Praise for Jorge Cruise and his *8-minute weight-loss plan*

'You won't have to count a single calorie, or even go to the gym.'
Daily Mirror

'Great results in less time than it takes to shower in the morning. If you have been procrastinating about starting an exercise programme, you have no more excuses.'
Kathy Smith, bestselling fitness author

'Diet guru Jorge Cruise has helped three million people lose weight with his revolutionary exercise and diet plan.'
Woman's Own magazine

'Jorge Cruise is the World's No. 1 online weight-loss specialist – favoured by Oprah Winfrey'
Evening Standard

'Jorge Cruise has answers that really work and take almost no time. I recommend them highly.'
Dr Andrew Weil, Director of the Program in Integrative Medicine, University of Arizona

'All you need is 8 minutes every day to sculpt a lean, toned body, putting an end to rushed lunchtime workouts and precious weekend hours spent in the gym'
Zest magazine

8 minutes in the morning® for

Lean Hips
and
Thin Thighs

Lose up to 10cm in less than 4 weeks!

8 minutes in the morning® for

Lean Hips and Thin Thighs

Lose up to 10cm in less than 4 weeks!

JORGE CRUISE

RODALE

This edition first published in the UK in 2005 by
Rodale International Ltd
7–10 Chandos Street
London W1G 9AD
www.rodale.co.uk

Printed and bound in the UK by CPI Bath using acid-free paper from sustainable sources.

1 3 5 7 9 8 6 4 2

A CIP record for this book is available from the British Library

ISBN 1-4050-7738-7

This paperback edition distributed to the book trade by Pan Macmillan Ltd

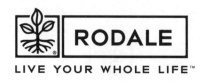

RODALE
LIVE YOUR WHOLE LIFE™

Notice

This book is intended as a reference volume only, not as a medical manual. The information given here is designed to help you make informed decisions about your health. It is not intended as a substitute for any treatment that may have been prescribed by your doctor. If you suspect that you have a medical problem, we urge you to seek competent medical help.

Mention of specific companies, organizations or authorities in this book does not imply endorsement by the publisher, nor does mention of specific companies, organizations or authorities in the book imply that they endorse the book.

Internet addresses and telephone numbers given in this book were accurate at the time the book went to press.

To all my online clients at JorgeCruise.com who sent me thousands of e-mails requesting that I write this book to help them get that special advantage to sculpt thinner thighs and hips faster. Enjoy!

Acknowledgements

First, I want to thank my 3 million (and growing) weight-loss clients at JorgeCruise.com whom I have had the privilege of coaching. Without all their feedback, insights and support, the Jorge Cruise weight-control brand would not be the success it is today.

I also must thank Oprah Winfrey, the lady who launched my career. She invited me to be a guest on her show in Chicago and introduced me to two people whose lives had changed because of my website. I will never forget that day. From that moment on, I knew that the Internet was a powerful resource that could change people's lives and bodies.

Heather, my wife, whom I love so much. Thanks again, baby doll, for being my source of love, balance, relaxation and fun. You have shown me what life is really about and how to enjoy it all. I love you with all my heart and soul.

To my mom, Gloria, who is my shining star in the sky that looks over me. To my dad, Mel, for being the man who inspired me by his original weight loss. To my sister, Marta, who shed over 30 pounds and is now helping the world with her books on dating, relationships and love. To my grandma Maria for showing me that at 92 years young resistance training can also add years to your life! To my grandpa George and grandma Dorothy who both passed away from being overweight…I promise to never forget the lesson from your passing about how essential it is to master you health before it's too late. I love you all.

To Phyllis McClanahan, my personal assistant and right hand. Thank you for keeping me focused and organized. You are priceless! Lisa Sharkey, my friend who has a heart of gold. To Bruce Barlean and the whole Barlean's family. Thanks for everything. To my buddy and great friend, Jade Beutler, and his family. To Ben Gage and his extraordinary negotiation and legal skills. To all my friends at Guthy-Renker, Harper-Collins, and Hay House. Thank you all so much!

A special big thank-you to Rodale Books for all their initial support with my 8 Minute books. In particular, Alisa Bauman for helping me convey my message, Kelly Schmidt for managing all the project details, Chris Rhoads for his extraordinary design skills, Jackie Dornblaser for getting me where I needed to go, and Stephanie Tade, who truly made this project possible. Also a special thank-you to Dana Bacher, Marc Jaffe, Steve Murphy, and the Rodale family.

To my stellar team at *Prevention* magazine for helping me get my weight-loss column out to 11 million readers each month. Rosemary Ellis, Michele Stanten and Robin Shallow, you are all the best!

Jan Miller, my literary agent, and Michael Broussard, her right arm, thank you for connecting me to the top people in the literary world. Jan, you are a gem. I look forward to a lifetime of great weight-loss books with you.

And finally, to my extraordinary and magical public relations team: Cindy Ratzlaff and Cathy Gruhn at Rodale, Mary Lengle at Spotted Dog Communications, and Arielle Ford and Katherine Kellmeyer at the Ford Group in San Diego. Thank you all so much from the bottom of my heart for your hard work, time, and efforts! Thank you, thank you, thank you!

Contents

Part 3: The Programme

Chapter 5

Bonus Chapter

Introduction

With Jorge's plan *I have lost 47 kg (105 lb) and more than 30 cm (12 in) off my thighs*. My 49th birthday present to myself was a professional picture taken of my granddaughter and me!

I feel like a new woman, I love being a young grandmother, and I'm looking forward to being 'Fifty and Fit'.

But I was not always this way. You see like many of you reading this, I have always been overweight. I have yo-yo'd on virtually every diet and have taken every over-the-counter diet aid. My weight has fluctuated my entire adult life – every time I lost weight I gained it, plus more!

In 1993, my family was in a tragic car crash. My eldest daughter broke her neck in two places, and my world as I knew it came to a screeching halt. I was driving when the accident happened, and the guilt was more than I could bear. Although my daughter never blamed me, I felt I needed to punish myself. As I have always been an emotional eater, I turned to food for comfort as it was always there for me. Sometimes the food felt very comforting, other times I used it as punishment.

Over the years, I have watched in admiration as my daughter turned this horrible experience into a reason to live on, and live happily. She once told me the accident happened for a reason and that it gave her a path in life. That night I kept thinking, 'Where is my path in life? To keep self-destructing?' At 1.5 m (5 ft) tall my weight ballooned up to over 90 kg (200 lb).

In 2001, I was blessed with a beautiful, healthy granddaughter, Talia. I was given a reason to be happy, to enjoy life, but I continued to knowingly eat unhealthily and gained more weight. I avoided being in pictures and videos with my granddaughter.

I remember clearly, when Talia was 11 months old, I was sitting on the floor watching her and

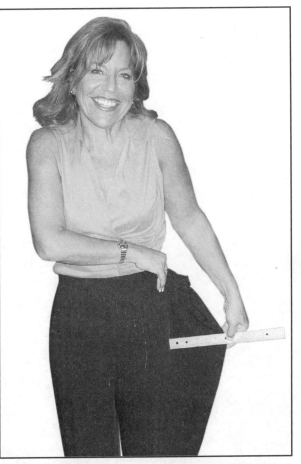

Nancy lost 30 cm (12 in) off her thighs!

thinking, 'I want her to be proud of me, not ashamed. I want to take her to the park; I want to be in pictures with her'. I remember tears welling up and that is when I started my new healthy life. As things are meant to be, it was soon after that I saw Jorge Cruise on TV. Since using his 8-minute technique, I have gone from 102 kg (225 lb) to 54 kg (120 lb).

I truly believe in Jorge's core philosophy that diets don't work and that the secret is to restore your resting metabolism by creating lean muscle. This plan will work for you…if you make the commitment.

My single most important tip to you right now so that you make a commitment that lasts is to believe in yourself. No matter what has happened in the past, no one can change your future but you. Find a blessing in your life, say 'thank you', and work each day to fulfil your goals. Thank you, Talia, for giving me a reason to be healthy and enjoy life… Thank you, Jorge, for giving me the tools to achieve my goals.

Nancy, JorgeCruise.com client

From the Desk of Jorge Cruise®

Dear Friend,

Welcome to my ALL-NEW *8 Minutes in the Morning for Lean Hips and Thin Thighs* book! I want to congratulate you and thank you for selecting me to be your coach. Together we are about to embark on the adventure of a lifetime.

You are probably wondering how in the next 4 weeks you will lose up to 10 cm (4 inches) from your hips and thighs in just 8 minutes a day. Well the answer is that there is a revolution going on in the field of weight loss. Aerobics and dieting are out. And resistance training is in. Experts agree the fastest way to lose weight is to build lean muscle tissue, which burns fat. The problem is that no one has time to workout.

Well, my *8 Minutes in the Morning for Lean Hips and Thin Thighs* programme has changed the rules. It will empower you to sculpt your hips and thighs at home and in just a few minutes a day.

So here's what I want you to do right now: first read Parts 1 and 2 of the book. It will show you how the programme works. Once you are done reading those areas, you will be ready to move on to Part 3. There you will start losing up to 10 cm (4 inches) in less than 4 weeks – in just 8 minutes a day. Enjoy!

JORGE CRUISE

The World's No. 1 online weight-loss specialist
www.jorgecruise.com

8 minutes

in the

morning® for

Lean Hips
and
Thin Thighs

Lose up to 10cm in less than 4 weeks!

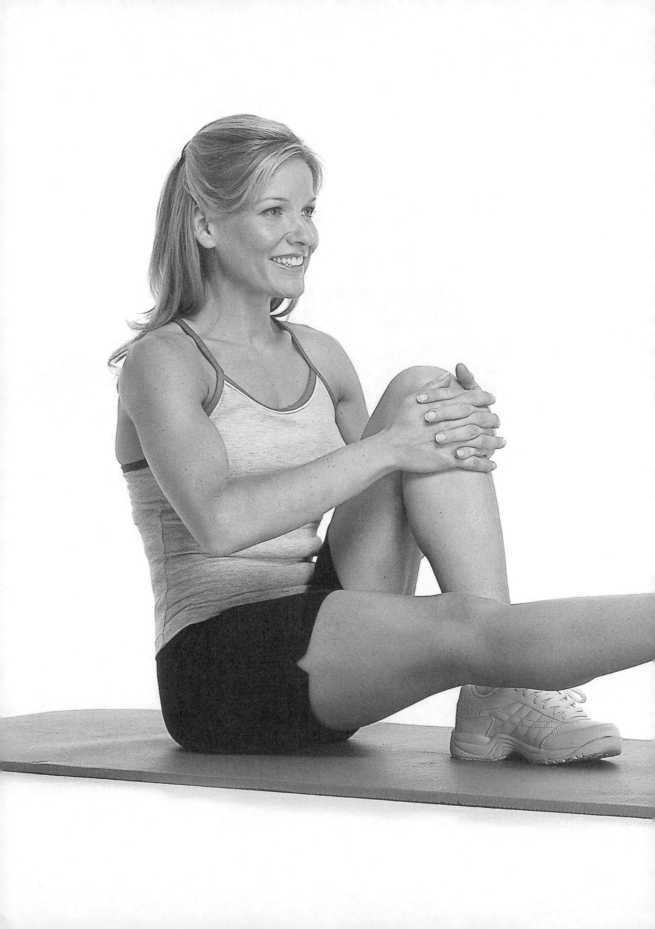

Part 1

Your Hips and Thighs

Chapter 1

Thin Thighs and Hips Await

Get Ready to Lose Up to 10 cm from Your No. 1 Trouble Zone in Just 8 Minutes a Day

8 minutes to firmer hips and thighs!

Welcome to *8 Minutes in the Morning for Lean Hips and Thin Thighs*. I'm so excited to bring you my latest 8 Minutes weight-loss solution, one specifically designed to address the number one trouble zone for women!

The fat that tends to accumulate along the thigh and hip area may very well be the most stubborn type of fat there is – and you probably don't need me to tell you that! That's why I'm so happy to tell you that no matter how stubborn the fat, you can burn it off.

your '8 minute' edge

8 Minutes in the Morning for Lean Hips and Thin Thighs will help you:

• Lose up to 10 cm (4 in) in less than 4 weeks

• Smooth away cellulite

• Boost your metabolism

• Allow you the convenience of doing it at home

And you don't need expensive food plans, pills, potions, or equipment. You don't need to spend hours at a gym. You don't even need to sweat and strain at home.

You need only commit to spending just 8 minutes each morning completing a set of targeted and effective moves. How can I promise to help you slim down your number one trouble spot in just 8 minutes a day when other programmes that took more time and more effort failed to yield results? Throughout the first few chapters of this book, you'll find the answer to that important question. But here's a sneak peek. *8 Minutes in the Morning for Lean Hips and Thin Thighs* is based on a revolution that is going on right now in the weight-loss industry. You see, aerobics – otherwise known as cardiovascular exercise – and dieting are out.

Experts now agree that to most efficiently shed fat, you must do resistance training to build lean muscle tissue. Lean muscle helps you to rev up your metabolism – no matter how sluggish. Train with me for just 8 minutes each morning and you'll boost your metabolism and sculpt your muscles, creating lean, sexy hips and thighs.

I believe resistance training is so important to your success that it is the cornerstone to *all* Jorge Cruise® weight-control plans. The Jorge Cruise® revolution will help you burn off the most stubborn fat deposits in your body and shape up the flabbiest muscles. Once you experience our simple 8-minute technique to restore your metabolism, I am confident you will *never* diet again.

the history of 8 minutes in the morning

I understand the struggle to lose weight and keep it off. I've struggled with weight as a child and young man. That struggle helped me create the Jorge Cruise® plan, which I published in *8 Minutes in the Morning*. That book – designed to help people lose up to 1 kg (2 lb) a week – quickly climbed the *New York Times* bestseller lists. I promptly followed up with my second book *8 Minutes in the Morning for Maximum Weight Loss*, designed to help those who wanted to lose more than 13 kg (30 lb).

As a result of the great success of both books, I appeared on numerous television programmes such as *Good Morning America*, CNN, *The View*, and *Dateline NBC*. It seemed every time I appeared on television, my website – www.jorgecruise.com – went crazy. As more and more people logged on to my site, I received more and more e-mails from people just like you, asking me to help them slim down their hips and thighs.

At the same time, my long-term clients who had already lost 10, 20, 30, or more pounds with my first two 8 Minutes programmes were telling me that they were ready to take the next step. They had lost most of the weight they wanted to lose. Yet they still wanted to give their hips and thighs some extra attention.

I responded as soon as I could. I designed an 8 Minutes pro-gramme that specifically targets the hip and thigh area. I tested it on my online clients over and over until I was completely confident that it would help all women get lean hips and thin thighs in just 8 minutes a day. The programme uses the Jorge Cruise® weight-loss formula and applies it specifically to the hips and thighs. I'm happy to tell you that anyone can use this supple-mentary programme to slim down the lower half – in just 8 minutes a day!

It doesn't matter whether you've lost weight with one of my other books or whether this is your first experience with the Jorge Cruise®

programme. Either way, you will experience fantastic results. If you haven't read my other books, that's okay. Everything you need to lose weight and slim down your hips and thighs is right here within the pages of this book.

the nature of hip and thigh fat

Many women tell me that every stray calorie seems to migrate to their hips and thighs. This is not a figment of their imaginations.

Before menopause, many women's bodies store excess fat predominantly in the hips and thighs, creating what's come to be known as the 'pear-shaped' body. Your body can easily mobilize this excess fat during pregnancy and breastfeeding, when the body needs as many as 1,000 extra calories a day. Fat storage in these sites dates back thousands of years, when it greatly helped certain cave-dwelling humans survive during times of drought and famine. Women who could easily store fat in their hips and thighs tended to be able to give birth and feed a baby during a drought, thus passing on their thigh-fat-storing genetics to future generations.

This is one reason why thigh fat is so difficult to get rid of. Genes left over from your cave-dwelling ancestors cause hormones and enzymes in your body to direct every extra calorie into waiting fat cells in your hips and thighs. For example, your levels of the female sex hormone oestrogen may be a tad higher than other women whose bodies don't store excess fat in these areas (or as much of it).

But there are ways to coax these fat cells in your thighs to release their contents, and to coax your muscle cells into burning it up! So don't despair.

the causes of cellulite

Besides excess fat in their thighs, many women complain to me about a certain type of fat known as cellulite. They tell me that no matter how much weight they lose, they can't seem to smooth out the tiny lumps of fat on their thighs. Indeed, some of the most slender women have cellulite. As many as 85 per cent of teenage girls have it.

Cellulite is created when fat manages to push its way through tiny holes in your connective tissue, the thick web of inter-woven fibres just underneath your skin. Strong and healthy connective tissue forms a tighter web of interwoven fibres, preventing fat from pressing its way through. Weak, unhealthy connective tissue, on the other hand, more easily stretches apart, allowing tiny fat pockets to poke through. Many factors can weaken your connective tissue, setting the stage for cellulite. They include:

High hormone levels. Women with higher-than-normal levels of the female hormone oestrogen tend to suffer more often from cellulite. Other than directing extra calories to fat cells in your thighs, oestrogen also weakens connective tissue. When oestrogen softens connective tissue around the womb, it makes childbirth possible. Unfortunately, oestrogen softens *all* of the connective tissue in your body, not just that around your womb.

Poor blood circulation. Usually, high oestrogen levels alone won't trigger cellulite to form. Many experts believe that you must also have poor blood circulation to your connective tissue, which tends to cause swelling. It is this swelling that stretches the connective tissue apart, allowing the fat to bulge through.

Fluid retention. Many people think that fluid retention takes place only in the abdomen. That's not true. It actually occurs all over your body, including your thighs. If you've ever pulled on a favourite pair of trousers and found them tight in the thighs on one day and loose on the next, you've experienced the ebb and flow of fluid retention. Any type of swelling in your thighs – particularly on a chronic basis – will stretch out and weaken connective tissue.

A frenzied lifestyle. Emotional stress has been shown to weaken connective tissue. My *8 Minutes in the Morning for Lean Hips and Thin Thighs* programme will help you smooth away cellulite in many ways. First, daily exercise will help to normalize your hormonal levels. This not only helps prevent cellulite, it will also help to prevent mood swings. Second, my Cruise Moves exercise programme will increase blood circulation to your thighs, helping to keep the connective tissue healthy. Better blood circulation will, in turn, help to remove excess fluid. Finally, as you shed fat in your hips and thighs, you'll have less of it to press against your connective tissue.

Frequently Asked Questions

Here are some questions that I often get from clients about their hips and thighs.

I've been doing lots of leg exercises, but it seems like my thighs are getting bigger and bigger. What's going on?

To slim down your thighs, you must build muscle all over your body to boost your metabolism to burn the fat. Doing lots of leg lifts will only build muscle in your legs, but won't burn the fat. As the muscle grows, your legs will grow. You must burn the fat to shrink the size of your thighs. My programme will help you to do just that.

It seems like every time I go on a diet, my upper body shrinks, but my lower body doesn't budge. Why does this happen?

The only way to shrink your lower body without shrinking your upper body is to stop dieting! Dieting sends your body into starvation mode. To help you survive the famine, your body preferentially burns fat in your upper body and conserves the fat in your lower body. The more often you diet, the more perverse this problem will become. The only way to burn fat in your lower body is to stop dieting and start strength training!

Everyone in my family has big thighs. Slimming my thighs is a hopeless battle, isn't it?

That couldn't be further from the truth. You may have inherited the tendency to store fat in your thighs from your parents, but that doesn't mean you can't burn the fat! Stick with me and you'll soon be a believer.

some good news and some bad news

Genetically speaking, there are two predominant body types. Some people gain fat in their lower bodies, creating the pear shape mentioned earlier. And still others tend to gain fat in their abdomens, creating what's known as an apple shape. (See my all-new *8 Minutes in the Morning for a Flat Belly*.)

Though you may have come to despise the fat on your hips and thighs, you should know that you have a major advantage over people who tend to gain it elsewhere. Research has shown over and over again that abdominal fat – and not hip and thigh fat – is particularly dangerous to your health. Abdominal fat more easily makes its way into your bloodstream, clogging your arteries. Thigh fat is much less likely to do so.

Now for the bad news. Thigh fat is a little harder to burn off than belly fat. You probably know this already. If you and a boyfriend, male friend, or husband have ever resolved to lose weight at the same time, you probably noticed that he had a much easier time dropping the weight in his belly than you did in your thighs.

Regardless, that doesn't mean you can't burn it off.

I know that women who have excess thigh fat are generally the most motivated to get rid of it. So I probably don't have to give you much of a pep talk to help motivate you toward your goal. Abdominal fat is easy to hide with a big sweater. Thigh fat, on the other hand, is almost impossible to hide. And summer can be a very difficult time for women. My female friends and online clients

Diane lost 10 cm (4 in)!

'I went from a size 16–18 trouser size to a size 12. I have lost 9 kg (21 lb) and feel so much better about myself. I feel better not only because I have dropped the weight but also because I feel I have so much more control over my life. I realize that I have choices and I am no longer a victim to food. I don't have to give up my favourite things; I just have them in smaller quantities. I am proud to say that I am over halfway to my goal and that I have learned other ways to cope with my stress than turning to food. Jorge has taught me some lifelong tools that I will always be able to fall back on in those difficult moments.'

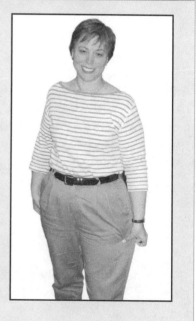

Diane dropped 3 sizes!

tell me that they hate wearing shorts and swimsuits because they hate revealing their legs. And they tell me that their trousers tend to hug too tightly in the thighs.

But you are going to change all of that! We are going to slim down those thighs and hips and smooth away that cellulite, creating a beautiful, sexy body from head to toe. Have you always wanted to wear those low-rise jeans but shunned them because they were too tight in the thighs? You'll be able to after finishing this *8 Minutes in the Morning for Lean Hips and Thin Thighs* programme. You'll be able to confidently bare your legs in shorts and swimsuits. Your thighs will no longer rub together when you walk.

And those are just the visual benefits. The muscles in your legs are some of the largest and strongest muscles in your body. Stronger leg muscles make your overall life feel so much more effortless. You'll walk with more confidence and a spring in your step. You'll be able to climb stairs without getting tired. And you'll be able to go on strenuous hikes – all because of your strong legs!

You will feel better about yourself from the inside out. And isn't that really what it's all about? Sure, you will look better. But you'll feel fantastic! **So promise me right now that you will make the commitment to sticking with the programme.** Promise me – and promise yourself – that you will find 8 minutes each day to complete your morning moves. Once you've made your promise, turn to chapter 2 to find out more about the magic of the 8 Minutes in the Morning programme.

Chapter 2

The Jorge Cruise® Revolution

Discover the Most Efficient Method for Slimming Your Hips and Thighs

rev up your metabolism

Now, let's take a closer look at the most important secret behind all of the Jorge Cruise® plans. To burn fat anywhere in your body – including your hips and thighs – you must restore your metabolism by creating new lean muscle tissue. Lean muscles provide the key that opens the lock on your metabolism, allowing you to turn up your metabolic furnace and burn fat all day long.

Remember in the previous chapter when I told you about a revolution in weight loss, one where aerobics and dieting are out and resistance training is in? Well, that revolution is based on this important fact about lean muscle tissue. Only resistance training, such as my unique Cruise Moves, helps create the lean muscle you need to rev up your metabolism and burn the fat. No other type of exercise provides such efficient and effective results.

the magic of lean muscle

Let's take a closer look at the amazing power of lean muscle tissue, starting with how it affects your metabolism.

Many factors affect your metabolism, and some are beyond your control. For example, some people are genetically gifted with fast metabolisms. These are those enviable people who do everything wrong: they eat huge servings of fattening foods and seem to never lift a finger. Yet, they never seem to gain an ounce. It seems no matter how much they eat, they remain as slim as a rail.

On the other hand, some people are genetically cursed with a slow metabolism. A left-over from years ago when calories were scarce, such a slow metabolism was helpful during times of famine. When food was scarce, someone whose body burned fewer calories and conserved the most fat tended to survive the longest.

Unfortunately, a slow metabolism doesn't help you much today. Today we are surrounded by calories in the form of fast food, frozen dinners and huge portions served up at restaurants. Food is abundant. And if you were genetically walloped with a slow metabolism, every stray calorie seems to make a beeline for your hips and thighs.

your '8 minute' edge

On the *8 Minutes in the Morning for Lean Hips and Thin Thighs* programme you will build lean muscle, which will help you:

• Speed up your metabolism

• Burn more calories 24 hours a day

• Shrink the size of your hips and thighs

Your age and gender also affect your metabolism. Men tend to burn more calories throughout the day than women. And as we age, certain hormonal changes also tend to slow the metabolism.

It's true that you can't change your genetics or age. But that doesn't mean your battle against hip and thigh fat won't be won. All of us have a very powerful metabolic weapon at our disposal, one that we can change for the better.

That weapon is *lean muscle tissue*.

Unlike fat, muscle is metabolically active tissue. Each half kilogram or pound of lean muscle tissue burns 50 calories a day.

That's why lean muscle is so important to your metabolism. It's the key to turning up your metabolic furnace and burning extra calories all day long.

the incredible shrinking muscle

Unfortunately, our lifestyles do not promote the creation or maintenance of lean muscle. Most of us sit during the vast majority of the day. We sit in our cars while on the way to work,

and then sit at a desk. Thanks to modern conveniences such as seated lawn mowers, self-propelled vacuum-cleaners, moving walkways, and escalators, we need not move much. The advent of electronic car windows means we no longer even need to roll these down ourselves. Food at the supermarket comes pre-chopped, so we don't need to use muscles in our hands and arms to turn a carrot into carrot slices. Each year, such labour-saving inventions become more and more prevalent – and we burn fewer calories as a result.

Due to lack of movement, our muscles tend to shrink with age. After the age of 20, most people lose about 2 kg (5 lb) of muscle per decade. By the age of 50, that amounts to 750 fewer burned calories a day – the amount of calories many people eat for breakfast and lunch. No wonder most of us tend to gain weight as we age!

Many people respond to creeping weight gain with dieting. But this couldn't be any more counterproductive. When you crash diet, your body goes into a survival mode, turning down your metabolism and turning up your appetite. It also tries to preserve your fat tissue by burning up your muscle tissue! This couldn't be more

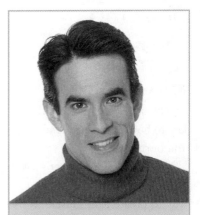

'Each half kilogram or pound of lean muscle tissue burns 50 calories a day.'

detrimental to your metabolism. You may succeed in losing the weight, but as soon as you go off the diet, it comes back – and then some. Worst of all, each time you diet, you slow your metabolism more and more.

You must reverse this destructive process by creating new lean muscle tissue. It's the only way to rev up your metabolism and slim down your hips and thighs for good!

how the jorge cruise® formula builds muscle

So you see, lean muscle is the key to boosting your metabolism and burning fat.

Now, let's take a closer look at the best and most efficient way to create lean muscle: resistance training. Though cardio-vascular activities such as running and walking maintain a certain amount of muscle, you'll get a much bigger return for your efforts with resistance training. And my targeted Cruise Moves will help you resistance train in the most efficient way possible.

Because of the way I've paired my Cruise Moves, you never need to rest during a session, which means that you never waste precious time between movements. Also, by working your muscles every day (with weekends off) you'll benefit from an exercise afterburn, boosting your metabolism a little more for the rest of the day after your sessions.

My programme takes just *8 minutes a day* to complete and that's key. Many people can motivate themselves at the beginning of a weight-loss pro-gramme to exercise for a half-hour or more. But that motivation usually wanes at some point. Does that sound familiar to you? Have you started and stopped fitness plans before?

the spot-toning myth

You may have heard very respected experts say that you can't spot tone. They say that you must learn to accept the shape of your body just the way it is. They say that you cannot shrink one area of your body and not another.

Well, I'm happy to tell you that the spot-toning caution is only half-true. Here's the truth: if you focus only on your thighs, for example, by doing hundreds of leg lifts, you probably won't slim down. Moving just one area of your body over and over doesn't result in fat burning in that one spot.

However, if you target your entire body – upper, middle, and lower – with certain resistance-training moves, you can boost your metabolism high enough that your body burns fat all day long. This will help burn fat all over your body, including your thighs. Doing resistance-training moves for your upper body will help fill out your weak area, helping to bal-ance your lower half. If you combine that with a healthy eating plan, you *will* shed the fat.

It's true that the fat in your thighs is the most stubborn type of fat there is. But that doesn't mean you can't burn it. An exciting study done at the University of Maryland and published in the prestigious *American Journal of Clinical Nutrition* showed that exercise and a healthy diet resulted in a 6.8-kg (15-lb) weight loss after 6 months. Though that may not sound like a lot of weight on the scale, know that these women were not extremely overweight to start with. And here's the real exciting news. The women were able to shrink their thigh circumferences by 4 per cent – the same amount as the rest of their bodies.

So, if you think that you lose weight every-where else in your body first – and in your thighs last – it may only be that you focused too much on calorie restriction and not enough on creating the lean muscle needed to boost your metabolism.

In order to stick with a programme, you must start a programme that easily fits into your life. You might struggle to find 30 minutes a day to exercise, but how about 8 minutes? I bet you can do that! Cruise Moves are designed to give you exactly what you need and no more. They will help you to fill out your shoulders and slim down your thighs, creating a balanced appearance.

You'll learn more about why the programme is so efficient in chapter 3.

In addition to 8 daily minutes of Cruise Moves, you will also get a delicious meal plan with essential muscle-making materials you'll need to create your new body. Remember: dieting slows the metabolism and shrinks muscle tissue. But overeating can be just as destructive as dieting, particularly if you overeat to soothe negative emotions.

My eating plan in chapter 4 will help you to avoid nutritional pitfalls. You'll learn how to eat nutritionally and *not emotionally*. You'll learn how to treat food as a tool for your body. Think of food as the tool that helps create lean muscle and boosts your metabolism.

a 2-step process

On the *8 Minutes in the Morning for Lean Hips and Thin Thighs* programme, you'll create lean muscle in two steps. Your first and most important step: 8 minutes of focused Cruise Moves each morning. These moves will create the lean muscle needed to boost your metabolism. They also will help to shape and tone your thighs, giving them a wonderful lean, enviable contour.

But to experience best results, you must combine your Cruise Moves with a second step: Eat Nutritionally, Not Emotionally. To create muscle, you must eat the materials to make muscle tissue. But you must not then overeat due to emotional stresses. If you overeat while doing your Cruise Moves, you'll hinder your success. Also, a healthy eating plan helps to support muscle growth and can also help boost your metabolism. You'll learn about this in chapter 4.

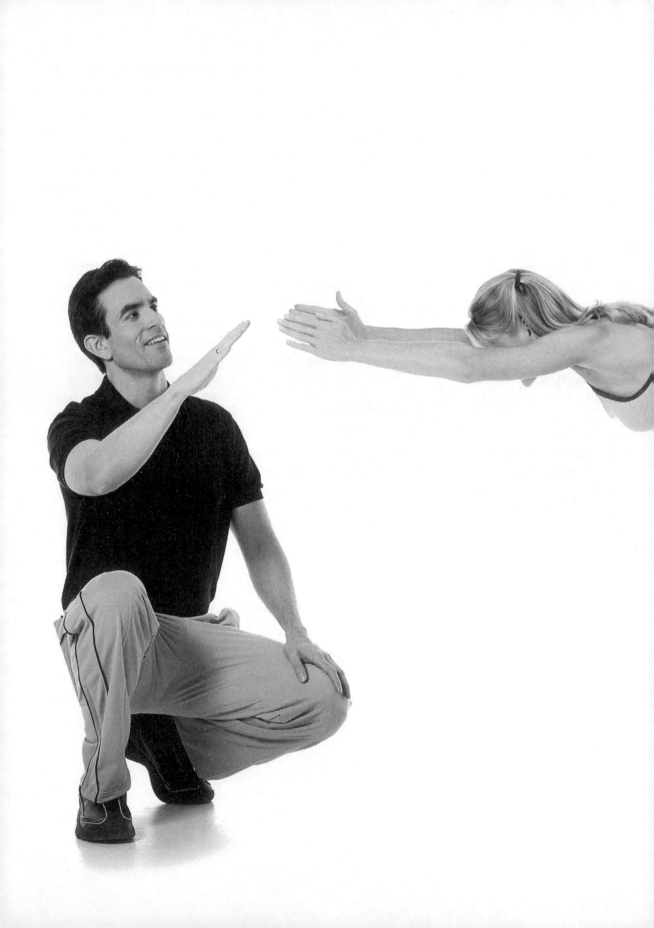

Part 2

How It Works

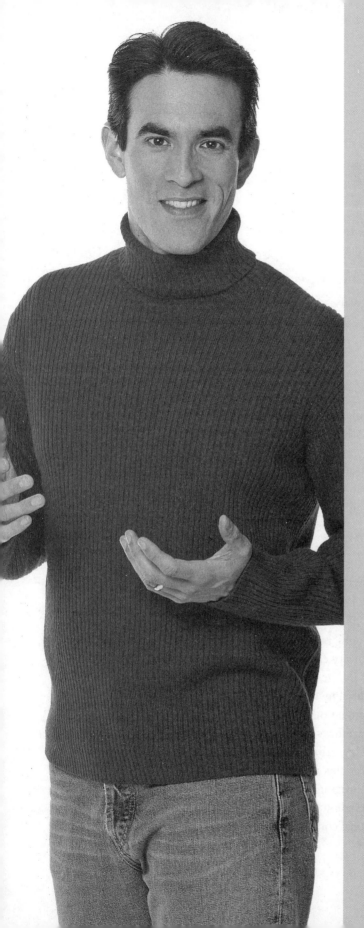

Chapter 3
Step 1

8 Minute Moves®

the magic 8 minute ingredient

Now that you understand why lean muscle is so important to your success, you're ready to find out how to create it. You're going to take your first step forwards on your journey to lean hips and thin thighs by learning about focused Cruise Moves.

These unique resistance-training exercises will help you to create the lean muscle needed to burn the fat in your lower body. Cruise Moves provide the magic 8 minute ingredient to help you thin down your thighs and create leaner hips. Cruise Moves are the most efficient, effective and convenient way to create lean muscle. They involve no aerobics and no trips to the gym. They take just 8 minutes each morning. And they're simple and easy to learn.

Cruise Moves will help you to sculpt beautiful long and lean muscle in your thighs and else-where. That lean muscle tissue will rev up your metabolism, helping you to incinerate excess fat. It will also help you tone and firm your hips and thighs,

along with the rest of your body. With the help of Cruise Moves, your thighs will appear longer, leaner and sexier. You'll want to show them off every-where you go!

your weekly schedule

In chapter 5, on pages 78 to 197, you will find three Cruise Moves programmes, ranging from very gentle to very challenging:

Level 1. The Cruise Moves for this level involve absolutely no equipment other than the chairs or pillows available in your home. They are very gentle and perfect for anyone starting a new exercise programme for the first time, including former professional couch potatoes.

Level 2. These Cruise Moves are slightly more challenging than Level 1. They, too, involve no equipment.

Level 3. The Cruise Moves at this level are the most are chal-lenging and involve the use of ankle weights, which are avail-able at any good sports shop.

No matter what your current fitness level, I suggest you start with Level 1. Follow Level 1 for 3 weeks before moving on to Level 2. Then do that programme for 3 weeks before moving on to Level 3. Three weeks will give your body the time it needs to adapt to the Cruise Moves. Within 3

your '8 minute' edge

Unlike other resistance-training programmes, your Cruise Moves sessions:

• Take only 8 minutes a day to complete

• Require minimal equip-ment

• Can be done in your own home, even while wearing your pyjamas.

weeks, you will have built enough muscle to allow you to tackle the next level with ease.

(*Note:* Level 1 may feel too easy for some of you right away. If you don't feel challenged by the exercises, move up to Level 2 after just 1 week with Level 1.)

For every level of the programme, you will follow the same schedule. (Consult 'Your Cruise Moves Schedule' on page 42.) You'll target your hips and thighs on Mondays, Wednesdays and Fridays with focused Cruise Moves for your lower body. On Tuesdays your Cruise Moves will target your upper body. On Thursdays they'll target your torso and calves.

Sometimes people ask me if they can skip the Cruise Moves on Tuesdays and Thursdays. 'My trouble zone is my lower half, not my upper half', they sometimes comment. I always tell them, as I am telling you right now, that you must create lean muscle *all over your body* – not just in your legs – in order to boost your metabolism high enough to see real results. Here's another important reason to tone your upper body: many pear-shaped women have very skinny shoulders and arms, which make their hips seem even wider. Resistance-training exercises will help to fill out your shoulders, creating

more balance between your shoulders and hips and helping to make your waist look smaller.

Here's another question that I often hear. Many people ask me whether they can speed their results by working their hips and thighs *every day*. The answer to that is a strong *NO*. You must give your muscles 48 hours to recover between sessions. That's when the true magic happens. During your time off from your hips and thighs routine, your muscles recover and grow stronger. If you work your hips and thighs every day – and you never give them a chance to recover – your muscles can never regenerate. Instead of speeding up your metabolism, you may instead slow it down. You'll end up feeling fatigued and you can even get injured.

The bottom line is that you achieve better results faster by targeting your trouble zone 3 days a week instead of 5 or more. Remember: when it comes to weight loss, less effort often produces more results! That's part of the Jorge Cruise® revolution.

a word about weekends

Each weekend you will get 2 days off from your Cruise

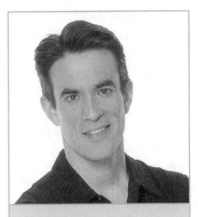

'You must create lean muscle *all over your body* to see real results.'

Moves. On Saturdays, I recommend that you spend your 8 minutes in the morning doing a set of stretches that will help lengthen your hip and thigh muscles. Don't misunderstand me. My Cruise Moves will help you to create long, lean muscles, not thick, bulky ones. However, these Saturday stretches will *accelerate* your results by helping to lengthen your leg muscles even more.

Whenever you stretch, you not only help increase your flexibility, but you also elongate your muscles. If you stretch often enough, your muscles will remain longer. And here's another good reason to stretch. It helps increase circulation to your muscles. This added circulation will help you to feel good, stretching away any tightness that may have developed during the week. It also may help reduce the appearance of cellulite. Stretching helps to improve the health of your connective tissue. Remember in chapter 1 when I told you about those tiny holes in connective tissue that allow small amounts of fat to bulge through, creating the bumpy appearance that we've come to call cellulite? Regular stretching helps your connective tissue stay healthy, closing up those gaps and preventing the fat from bulging through.

If you already have a set of stretches that you love to do, that's great. Go ahead and do them. If not, you'll find my favourite stretches in the bonus chapter on page 199.

Each Sunday, you have the day off. You have no stretches and no Cruise Moves in the morning. I suggest that you use Sundays to record your progress: weigh yourself and measure your hip and thigh circumferences.

Try to use Sundays as a true respite from the week. Make it your time to relax and rejuvenate. Many of my clients tell me that they like to set aside some time each Sunday to plan and prepare for the week ahead. You might chop up some veggies to use during the week for lunch or plan your dinner menus and make sure you have healthy food on hand. Do whatever you need to do to make sure your week goes smoothly – you'll increase your chances of sticking to your morning moves and your Cruise Down Plate, which you'll learn about in chapter 4.

the format for each day

No matter what, the format for your day will be the same. You will wake up and do whatever you need to do to ready yourself for your morning moves. Some of my clients tell me that after a trip to the bathroom, they like to splash some water on their faces, drink a glass of water and brush their teeth. After that, they are ready to move.

Each morning during the week you will find four Cruise Moves. **You will do each move for 1 minute and then move on to the next move. Once you have finished all four moves, you will repeat each move one time for 1 minute each – for a total of 8 minutes.**

It's that easy.

How can you complete a session so quickly? I've strategically paired your Cruise Moves so that you will always be working opposing muscle groups. For example, when you target your inner thigh, your outer thigh gets to rest. When you target your outer thigh, your inner thigh gets to rest. I call this *Active Rest Moves*®. That way, you never need to rest between moves. There's no wasted time on the 8 Minutes programme. You simply transition from move to move for 8 minutes. It's a focused programme, and it works!

your cruise moves schedule

Here's what you will be doing each day on the *8 Minutes in the Morning for Lean Hips and Thin Thighs* programme.
monday: Hips and Thighs
tuesday: Chest, Upper Back, Biceps, Triceps
wednesday: Hips and Thighs
thursday: Belly, Lower Back, Shoulders, Calves
friday: Hips and Thighs
saturday: Muscle Lengthening and Stretching
sunday: Day Off – Assess Your Progress

how you'll address your trouble zone

Now here's where things get really exciting. If you've tried to slim down your hips and thighs in the past, you may have noticed that particular exercises seem to make your hips and thighs larger! That usually happens when you solely focus on just one area of the thigh.

Well, you'll be happy to hear that there is a mix of moves in this book. These moves are sorted into four thigh zones.

Here are the four zones you will target 3 days a week.

Inner thighs. The muscles along your inner thighs are collectively known as your adductors, because they are responsible for 'adducting' or pulling your legs in toward the centreline of your body. Toning these muscles will not only help keep your inner thighs from jiggling, but also will help to pull your inner thighs closer to your thigh bone, shrinking their appearance and preventing them from rubbing together when you walk.

Front of the thighs. The muscles along the front of your thighs are collectively called your quadriceps and hip flexors. They help you to extend and lift your leg forward.

Outer thighs and hips. The muscles that are on your outer thighs and hips are collectively called your abductors because they 'abduct' or lift your leg away from the centreline of your body. (Think of the quintessential leg lift.) Along your hips, the most important abductor is the gluteus medius. Toning this muscle, along with your other abductors, will help smooth away saddlebags. These muscles also help to hold your kneecap in place, so training them will help to prevent knee pain.

Backs of the thighs and rear end. A number of different muscles make up the backside of your leg. Along the back of your thigh are a group of muscles called your hamstrings. In your buttocks, there's the gluteus maximus. Your hamstrings and gluteus maximus work together to help lift your leg back behind your torso. Your hamstrings also help you to bend your knee. Toning your hamstrings will help smooth out the back of your thigh and reduce the appearance of cellulite. It also will help to provide separation between your thigh and bottom. Toning your gluteus will help lift your bottom.

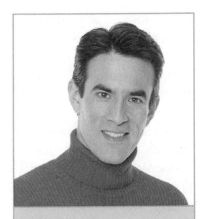

'When it comes to resistance training, less time often produces more results!'

why you should move in the morning

Once you understand the power of exercising in the morning, you'll never go back to afternoon or evening workouts.

First, when you move in the morning, you're more likely to feel good for the rest of the day. You feel stronger, more energized and less stressed. In a study at the University of Leeds in England, researchers found that women who exercised in the morning reported less tension and greater feelings of contentment for the rest of the day than those who didn't exercise in the morning. When you do your Cruise Moves, you send a signal to your pituitary gland to release endorphins, your body's natural feel-good chemicals. The more endorphins you have in your bloodstream, the better you feel. Thanks to morning exercise, you will be able to handle stress better no matter what happens in your day.

But that's not all. Moving in the morning also helps you to shed fat faster than moving at other times of the day. When you first wake up, your metabolism is sluggish because it has slowed down during sleep. But when you exercise, your metabolism increases. By doing your Cruise Moves first thing in the morning, you boost your metabolism when it's normally at its slowest. You're also better able to build lean muscle when you move in the morning. Resting levels of testosterone, the body's primary muscle-building hormone, are the highest in the morning. This suggests that the muscle-creating potential of resistance training may be at its peak before noon.

In short, you burn more calories when you exercise in the morning, making better use of your exercise time.

Finally, moving in the morning

just sleep on it

Many of my clients give me a funny look when I tell them that an **extra hour** of sleep at night could help them to lose weight faster. Here's why sleep is so important to your success. It's during deep, stage 4 sleep that your body repairs and regenerates itself. During stage 4 sleep your body secretes growth hormone, a protein used to repair muscles and injured tissues. If you don't spend enough time in stage 4 sleep, this important body repair process doesn't fully complete itself.

In fact, researchers suspect that people who have chronic pain syndromes like fibromyalgia don't spend enough time in stage 4 sleep. In experiments done in the 1970s, it took just a week of light sleeping – where people were not allowed to enter stage 4 sleep – before muscle aches and pains popped up.

Other research has found that getting just 1 hour too little of sleep can lower levels of the hormone testosterone. Though more abundant in men, both men and women have this hormone, important in the muscle-creating process. When you don't have enough testosterone, it throws off your muscle-to-fat ratio, promoting fat storage and hindering muscle development.

Not getting enough sleep can also cause depression and bad moods, which can lead to overeating. It also lowers your immunity, which can lead to colds that force you to skip your Cruise Moves sessions. Finally, when you go to bed on time, you're more likely to get out of bed on time – in time to do your Cruise Moves.

Surveys show that only about ⅓ of people sleep at least 8 hours. Promise me that you will make sleep a priority. Turn off the TV and head to bed at a reasonable hour. Your body and thighs will thank you.

helps you to stay consistent. Have you ever *planned* to exercise in the afternoon or evening only to skip those plans because something else came up? That usually doesn't happen first thing in the morning. Simply put, your morning is *your* time. It's the easiest time to control. You can roll out of bed, do your moves and have some extra time just for you.

Later in the day, distractions will come up. Your spouse, your children, your job, or an emergency will interrupt your plans and force you to put your Cruise Moves on hold. Research shows that only 25 per cent of evening exercisers consistently do their exercise routines, compared to 75 per cent of morning exercisers. The bottom line is that when you commit to exercising in the morning, you bypass excuses and shed weight faster because you are more consistent.

8 minutes is all you need

So now that you understand how Cruise Moves will slim down your hips and thighs, I ask you to promise yourself that you will commit to 8 minutes each morning. That's all you need – just 8 minutes. I'm not asking for 20 or 30 or 45. *Just 8 minutes.* So set your alarm to wake you 8 minutes earlier and start going to bed earlier at night. And then turn to chapter 4 to find out about the important second step in your journey to lean hips and thin thighs.

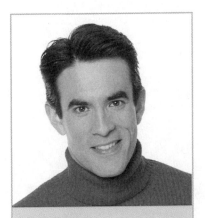

'When you commit to exercising in the morning, you bypass excuses and shed weight faster.'

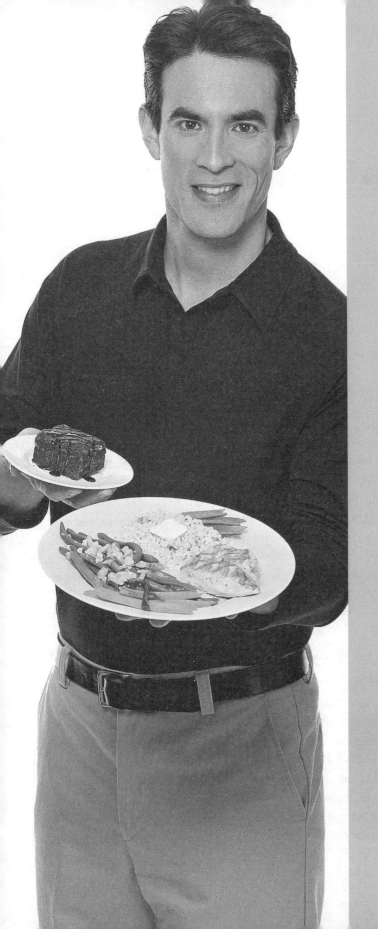

Chapter 4
Step 2

Eat Nutritionally,
Not Emotionally®

the simplest eating system

You just learned about your first step for your journey to leaner hips and thinner thighs. Now you're ready to learn about the second step to weight-loss success. You'll learn how to optimize muscle creation with a healthy eating plan that provides your body with the muscle-making materials to make your new body!

Remember when I told you in chapter 2 that eating too little can be just as destructive as eating too much? Well, I've developed the perfect system to help you eat the right foods in the right amounts. This will not only optimize muscle creation, but it will also help boost your metabolism and eliminate the cravings that can lead to

your '8 minute' edge

By eating nutritionally – and not emotionally – you will be able to:

- Optimize muscle growth
- Boost your metabolism
- Eliminate cravings
- Increase your energy
- Burn more fat

overeating and self-sabotage. I call this system the *Cruise Down Plate*®. It's a very simple eating plan that will help you to automatically eat the right foods in the right portions. Also, the plate will help you to continue to eat the foods you love as well as a few crucial foods that will help turn down your appetite and turn up your fat-burning furnace.

how the plate works

The Cruise Down Plate is really very simple. For breakfast, lunch and dinner, place your food on a standard 23-cm (9-in) dinner plate. Fill half the plate with vegetables (or fruit at breakfast) and the other half with equal portions of carbohydrate and

protein foods, along with a teaspoon of fat. If you are still hungry, you can have another plate of vegetables. It's that easy!

I know it sounds too simple to be true. But it really works.

When you follow the Cruise Down Plate, you will eat the right balance of carbohydrate, fat and protein. This is so important, particularly to building lean muscle tissue. Your muscles are made of protein and they repair and rebuild themselves with the protein from the food you eat. In addition, eating some protein at every meal will help to turn down hunger, as protein takes longer to digest than carbohydrate.

The fat on your plate is also very important. Too often, people who are trying to lose weight try to get their fat calories down to zero. They have heard that fat contains more calories per gram than carbohydrate or protein and that the body most efficiently shuttles fat into fat cells. However, this isn't completely accurate!

Only some fats are bad for you. They include the saturated

THE CRUISE DOWN PLATE®

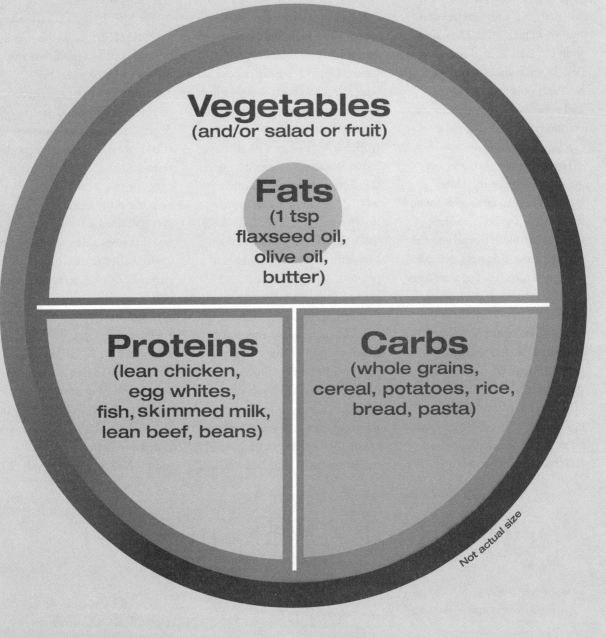

Vegetables
(and/or salad or fruit)

Fats
(1 tsp
flaxseed oil,
olive oil,
butter)

Proteins
(lean chicken,
egg whites,
fish, skimmed milk,
lean beef, beans)

Carbs
(whole grains,
cereal, potatoes, rice,
bread, pasta)

Not actual size

Follow one simple rule: fill half of a standard 23-cm (9-in) plate with vegetables and the other half with equal portions of carbohydrates and protein foods, along with a teaspoon of fat. It's that easy!

and hydrogenated fats found in animal products and fried and processed foods. These are the fats that clog your arteries and lead to weight gain. They are found in fatty animal products (whole milk, cheese, fatty cuts of beef and pork) as well as fried and processed foods (fast foods, commercially baked goods, crackers and chips).

However, other fats are very good for your health. They include essential fatty acids found in flax seeds and flax products (such as flax meal, flax oil and flax supplements), fish, nuts, avocados, olives and olive oil. You need some dietary fat to boost your mood, help your body digest important vitamins, and make hormones. Fat also helps you feel satisfied, helping you to enjoy eating and stop before it's too late. A wealth of research has now found that the key to weight loss is cutting back on saturated and hydrogenated fats and eating more essential fatty

acids. Flax seed oil is my favourite 'weight-loss' fat as it's very rich in essential fatty acids.

Here's another way the Cruise Down Plate helps fuel weight loss. The vegetables on your Cruise Down Plate are packed with fibre. You body digests fibre slowly, helping to turn down your hunger. Because your body must work harder to digest high-fibre foods, it wastes calories during the digestive process. In other words, your body burns more calories to break down high-fibre foods than it does to break down low-fibre foods such as mashed potatoes or white bread.

In addition to following the Cruise Down Plate, I suggest that you pay careful attention to your liquid calories. Many people drink more calories – often in the form of soft drinks – than they realize. Also, beverages that contain alcohol and caffeine create toxins that get trapped in the fat tissue in your body. This

can create fluid retention where you tend to store the most fat – your hips and thighs.

You don't have to completely give up soft drinks, alcohol and caffeine, but I suggest that you make careful choices. For example, instead of coffee, you might switch to green tea or decaf. Green tea not only contains less caffeine than coffee, but research has also shown that it contains special substances that help boost the metabolism. If you love soft drinks, hold yourself to two diet ones a day. If you like to unwind after work with an alcoholic drink, you might dilute it. For example, try a wine spritzer instead of pure wine.

Finally, I suggest you optimize your water intake by drinking eight 220 ml (8 fl oz) glasses of water a day. About 60 per cent of your muscles are made up of water and your metabolism needs water in order to burn body fat for energy. Dehydration can slow fat

the thigh-thickening fats

Avoid these types of fat:

- Processed foods containing 'partially hydrogenated fats'
- Margarine
- Shortening
- Fried foods

- Fatty cuts of beef and pork
- Chicken and turkey skins
- Butter
- Egg yolks

the thigh-friendly fats

Eat more of these fats:

- Flaxseed oil and ground flax seeds (more on flax at www.jorgecruise.com/flax)
- Extra-virgin olive oil and olives
- Avocados and guacamole
- Fatty cold-water fish such as salmon
- Nuts, especially almonds
- Almond butter
- Rapeseed (canola) oil

burning. It also can sap your energy, making you too tired to do your Cruise Moves. Water also contains oxygen. For muscle tissue to burn fat, it needs oxygen to help convert fat into energy. When you drink water, you improve your oxygen levels, improving your metabolism. Finally, water also helps to flush toxins out of the body and reduce bloating, which can improve circulation to your legs, reducing the appearance of cellulite and helping with fat burning.

You can meet your fluid requirements either with plain water – preferable because it has no calories – or with other non-caffeinated drinks and high-water-content foods such as soup, fruits and vegetables.

the three rules of the plate

To make the Cruise Down Plate work for you, you must follow three simple rules:

1. Eat breakfast within 1 hour of rising.

2. Eat every 3 hours.

3. Stop eating 3 hours before bed.

Here's why. Let me start with breakfast. To keep your metabolism up, you must eat your first meal within 1 hour of rising. As you sleep, your body is not getting any food and consequently turns down your metabolism. When you awake, you want to kick your metabolism back into high gear as soon as possible. If you don't eat within 1 hour of waking, your body will protect the most precious calorie-rich tissue in your body that it will need to survive during a famine: body fat. It turns down your metabolism even more and begins to cannibalize muscle tissue instead of fat tissue.

So, if you skip breakfast, you just end up damaging your efforts.

This is the same reasoning behind why you should eat every 3 hours.

Frequent meals will help keep your metabolism running smoothly for the rest of the day. The key is to eat five mini-meals throughout the day, each one separated by 3 hours. In other words, this means you might eat breakfast at 7.00 a.m., then have a snack at 10.00 a.m., then eat lunch at 1.00 p.m., then a snack at 4.00 p.m., and finally dinner with a treat at 7.00 p.m. This is a perfect eating schedule, and I strongly recommend you follow it closely.

Finally, let's talk about why you should stop eating 3 hours before bed. When the sun goes down each day, your body's temperature begins to drop and vital functions like heartbeat and breathing begin to slow down, preparing you for sleep. If you can eat in a way that supports this natural rhythm, you will ensure that your body gets a full night's rest.

If you eat close to your sleep time, you take too much food to bed with you, and your digestive system keeps you awake as it breaks down your food. Though you may actually be able to fall asleep, you won't sleep deeply as your body digests. And you need *deep* sleep in order for your body to truly rest and recover.

If you eat too late at night, your body spends its energy on digestion rather than on repairing and firming your lean muscle tissues. Your goal is to make sure that you recuperate

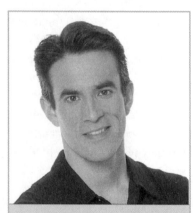

'Never give up, surrender, or quit.'

during sleep rather than waste your rest on digestion. I promise you will feel more energized and alive when you wake!

the dangers of emotional eating

Many people can easily follow the Cruise Down Plate and never feel tempted to overeat. But I know that some of you will need a little extra help, particularly those of you who tend to eat for emotional rather than physical reasons.

What is emotional eating? It's any time you eat when you are not physically hungry. Emotional eating is the number one cause of self-sabotage. Before they came to me for coaching, many of my clients told me that they turned to food whenever they felt distress in their lives. They ate when they were happy, sad, nervous – you name it. For them, food had become a crutch that they used to soothe themselves.

To stop the self-sabotage and end emotional eating, you must learn to discern between nutritional hunger and emotional hunger. Nutritional hunger is a biological need. It's all about eating to provide your body with the building materials it needs to stay healthy and build lean

muscle. **Emotional hunger often comes from a lack of support, comfort and warm nurturing from people.** Only when you replace food with the support from friends and family will you be able to step off the emotional eating roller coaster.

In my last book, *8 Minutes in the Morning for Maximum Weight Loss*, I created a powerful technique called The People Solution. It gave my clients strong protection from emotional eating. Since the publication of that book, I've heard many success stories from readers who tried it and loved it. The People Solution teaches you how to use the power of people to support you and replace the need and comfort from food. It includes three key tactics:

1. Become your own greatest friend. Too often, people have a love-hate relationship with their bodies. Yet to experience success, you must respect your body and treat it as the greatest gift you've ever received. Only when you respect your body will you firmly commit yourself to your Cruise Moves and feed your body healthy foods. To become your own greatest friend, I suggest you create a 'Power Pledge Poster'. On the poster, write the phrase, 'My current body is the most precious gift I have ever been given'. Underneath that, write the positive consequences of believing that statement. For example, you might write, 'I will treat my body as a top priority' or 'I will feed my body properly'. Then, underneath those consequences, write 10 sentences that describe why your body is a precious gift. For example, you might write, 'My body helps me to get to where I need to go'. I encourage you to create your own Power Pledge Poster. After you do so, photocopy it three times and post it in three spots in your house or at work where you will see it often.

2. Establish a support team. Create a support network of seven people who will help motivate you to stick to the programme. Your inner team can include family, colleagues and good friends. You should choose people that allow you to feel comfortable communicating your feelings. Three of these people should be 'e-mail' friends, people you can e-mail at any time of the day or night when you feel you might be about to slip up. Three others should be phone friends, people who will agree to literally be on call in case you need support. One person should be an accountability friend, someone you can meet with once a week to go over the specifics of the programme along with your challenges and breakthroughs.

3. Expand your inner team. In addition to picking seven people you already know to help support your efforts, you will continually add more and more people to your inner team. You might do that by joining or starting a weight-loss book group or by going online to JorgeCruise.com and meeting millions of Cruisers who are taking the same journey as you!

In *8 Minutes in the Morning for Maximum Weight Loss*, I include many more specifics about The People Solution. However, you now know enough to get started. If you'd like more tips on implementing The People Solution into your life, I suggest you pick up a copy of *8 Minutes in the Morning for Maximum Weight Loss*.

safety in a belt

Since the publication of *8 Minutes in the Morning for Maximum Weight Loss*, I found that although The People Solution certainly helped my clients to eliminate nearly all cases of emotional eating, some people still encountered emergency emotional eating situations, situations that I like to call Doughnut Moments.

To help my clients completely immunize themselves from even the most tempting of temptations, I created The Safety Belt System.

It works like this. Think about driving down the road in a really safe car, such as a Volvo. You feel secure because you know the car was made specifically to protect you and the passengers in case of an accident. Were you to get in an accident, the Volvo's state-of-the-art frame would absorb the impact, keeping your body safe.

But even in a Volvo, you wouldn't drive down the road without your seatbelt, right? That's the same principle here. My People Solution provides you with the safe car. It will help to reduce the emotional impact along the road of life. But you also want to be safe in case of sudden accidents that may toss you out of the car. You'll need a seatbelt to keep you safely behind the driver's seat of healthy eating and weight loss.

My Safety Belt System provides you with a strong set of seatbelts to help you overcome any situation that may drive you to eat emotionally. Just as racing-car drivers have multiple seatbelts to keep them extra safe on the road, you'll have multiple seatbelts to keep you extra safe in the kitchen, restaurants, cafeteria, and whenever you find yourself around food.

The Safety Belt System

With the help of millions of online and personal clients, I've come up with the following five 'seatbelts' to help you prevent random acts of overeating.

Belt Number 1
The Safety Bracelet

Take a small child's belt or even a dog collar and attach it to your handbag or wallet. That way, whenever you must reach for money to buy food that doesn't support your goal, you will see the belt and remember your commitment to yourself.

'My safety bracelet is always with me,' says Lisa, one of my clients. 'I use it like an indicator light to remind me to stop before I eat something that I will regret later.'

Belt Number 2
Throw It Out and Shout

Researchers have found that we humans are genetically programmed to eat all of the food that we see. That's why, if you eat ice cream straight from the container or chips straight from the bag, you always eat more than you intend. It's also why many people tend to overeat at buffet-style restaurants.

To overcome such 'see food' temptations, one of my clients, Cariann, has come up with this unique strategy. She allows herself to eat the foods she loves and craves. She knows, as I've told her, that if she forbids herself to eat a certain food, she will crave it even more and eventually binge on it. However, to keep herself from going overboard on delicious treats, she buys the treat, measures out the portion that she'll allow herself and then she throws the rest away.

'When you have thrown out the remainder away, shout "I'm thin!" or "Control!" or simply "Yahoo!"' she suggests. 'If you take the remainder of the bag with you into the car or you keep holding it, you will probably eat all of it.'

Belt Number 3
See and Be Bookmark

Take a photo of yourself at your heaviest and another photo of yourself at your skinniest (or some other inspiriting photo) and make a bookmark out of them. Paste them together back to back and then take them to a stationers for lamination. Keep one in this book and use others in any other book or magazine that you tend to pick up throughout the day to help remind yourself of your goal! Look at your bookmark any time you feel the urge to eat when you are not hungry.

Belt Number 4
The Olf Factor

Have you ever turned your nose up at a food primarily because of the way it smelled, regardless of how it tasted? Your sense of smell, also called your olfactory sense, is very powerful and can affect how much you enjoy your food.

That's why I suggest you mentally conjure up a disgusting smell whenever you find yourself craving a food when you are not truly hungry. Often, just thinking about a bad smell is enough to turn off your emotional appetite for a certain food. And just as getting a bad stomach upset after eating a certain food will make you avoid that food, this smell association will make you avoid certain foods.

My client Liz suggests that you 'Think of a smell so bad that it makes you feel sick, such as the smell of your kid's stinky nappy or the smell of dead, rotting fish or the smell of rotten meat on a hot day. Pick whatever smell makes you the sickest in that crucial moment when you are about to eat when you are not truly hungry.'

Belt Number 5
The Home Run

This is so simple yet so powerful. I recommend that you set www.jorgecruise.com as your home page on your computer at work and your computer at home. Whenever you go onto the Internet, my site will come up and you'll get a great reminder of your success. Every day I post an inspiring quote that will help motivate you to stay on track. You can also ask me questions or go to any of the chat rooms or discussion boards for extra support. As one of my clients says, 'When I am at work, I just turn my computer on and see Jorge's face and I feel like he is watching me – and I wouldn't sabotage myself if he was physically here with me!'

Renee lost 9 cm (3½ in)!

'I lost 5 cm (2 in) in one thigh and 4 cm (1½ in) in the other (my right thigh was larger than my left thigh to start with) and I have dropped 20 kg (44 lb)!

I loved these exercises because that is the area where I needed the most toning. It is a family genetic factor that I carry a lot of my weight in my thighs, and I was happy to shed those inches!!!

I'm in my seventies now, and I am wearing the same size that I wore in my thirties. I love that I don't have to hide behind baggy clothes any more.'

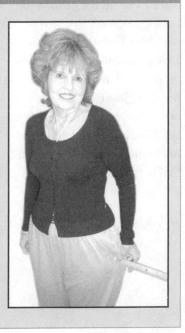

Renee lost 20 kg (44 lb)!

sample meals for easy eating

If you're still not quite sure how to use the Cruise Down Plate, you'll find everything you need to know right here.

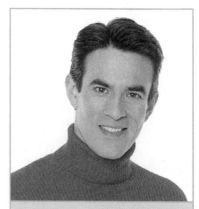

simple and delicious

For help on figuring out how to place foods on the plate in the correct portions, I've started you off with a few sample Cruise Down Plate meals. The photos on pages 57–60 will help you get on track. Just remember: these are optional samples. To follow the Cruise Down Plate, you need only follow one simple rule: fill half the plate with vegetables and the other half with equal portions of carbohydrate and protein foods, along with a teaspoon of fat. And if you are still hungry, have another plate of vegetables. It's that easy!

Use these photos for ideas and inspiration. And don't forget that you can spice up all of these meals with any seasonings or condiments from my 'freebies' list on pages 66–67. Enjoy, and eventually you'll be creating your own delicious Cruise Down Plates in the right portions for weight loss. For even more help on ensuring you fill your plate with the right portions, check out my food lists on pages 61–67.

'If you are still hungry, have another plate of vegetables.'

critical secrets

Follow one simple rule for the Cruise Down Plate: fill half your plate with vegetables, a quarter of your plate with carbohydrate foods, a quarter of your plate with protein foods, and use one teaspoon of fat.

Sample 1

Breakfast Veggie omelette (6 egg whites mixed with lots of veggies); ½ bagel with 1 teaspoon reduced-fat cream cheese; 115 g/4 oz juice-packed pineapple chunks

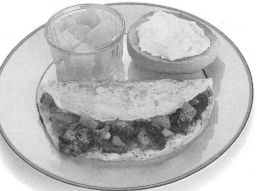

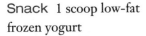

Snack 12 cashews

Lunch Sandwich (2 slices of wholemeal bread, 60 g/2 oz turkey, 1 slice of lean bacon, lettuce, sliced tomatoes); ⅛ avocado; 240 ml (8 fl oz) vegetable soup

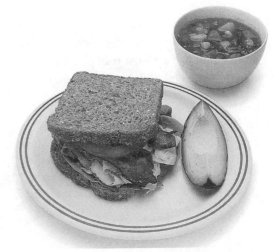

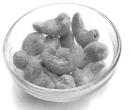

Snack 1 scoop low-fat frozen yogurt

Dinner 'Fried' chicken (90 g/3 oz chicken rolled in breadcrumbs and baked); 115 g/4 oz mashed potatoes with 1 teaspoon olive oil; steamed veggies

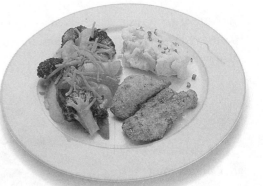

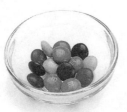

Treat ¼ small bag M&M's

Sample 2

Breakfast ½ muffin spread with 1 tablespoon almond or peanut butter; 1 sliced apple

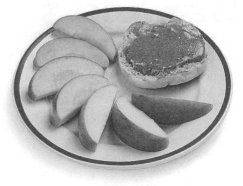

Snack Low-fat cereal bar

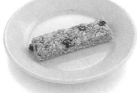

Lunch Sandwich (90 g/3 oz canned tuna mixed with 1 tablespoon reduced-calorie mayonnaise and stuffed into half a 15-cm/6-in pitta); lettuce and tomatoes; 240 ml (8 fl oz) tomato soup

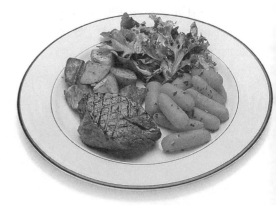

Snack 2 tablespoons pumpkin seeds

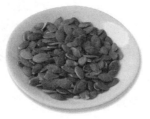

Dinner 90 g/3 oz lean steak served with 115 g/4 oz roasted red potatoes; steamed carrots; mixed green salad with 1 teaspoon flaxseed oil

Treat 1 chocolate-coated after-dinner mint

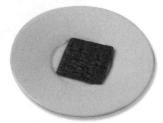

Sample 3

Breakfast 170 g/6 oz low-fat yogurt mixed with 60 g/2 oz sugar-free muesli, 145 g/5 oz mixed berries, and 6 slivered almonds

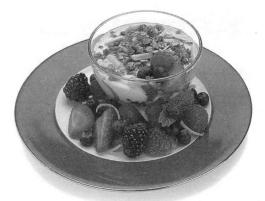

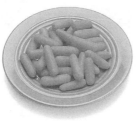

Snack 230 g/8 oz baby carrots

Lunch Hot dog with 1 tablespoon mustard and ketchup on bun; mixed green salad with 1 teaspoon olive oil

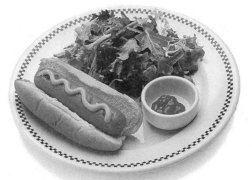

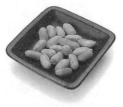

Snack 20 peanuts

Dinner 1 square spinach lasagne; mixed green salad with 1 teaspoon flaxseed oil and chopped fresh garlic

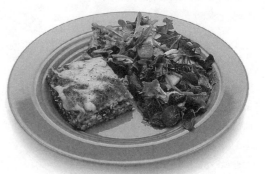

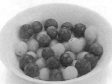

Treat 115 g/4 oz frozen seedless grapes

Sample 4

Breakfast 3 slices of extra-lean or 2 slices lean bacon; 1 slice of granary bread; 125 g (4½ oz) sliced strawberries, 60 g (2 oz) low-fat yogurt

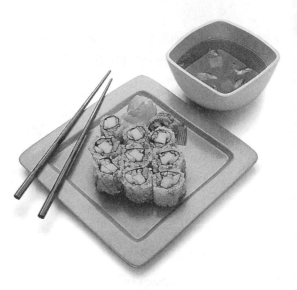

Snack celery sticks, filled with 1 tablespoon peanut butter

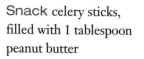

Lunch 9 small pieces of sushi (rice, crabmeat, cucumber, avocado, seaweed); 240 ml (8 fl oz) miso soup

Snack 2 tablespoons raisins

Dinner Taco (60 g/2 oz lean minced beef, 15-cm/6-in corn tortilla, 30 g/1 oz low-fat/fat-free grated cheese, shredded lettuce, diced tomatoes, salsa); mixed green salad with 1 teaspoon flaxseed oil

Treat 1 miniature chocolate bar

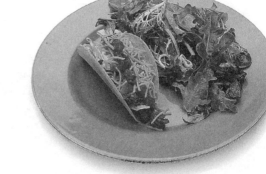

cruise down plate optional food lists

As I shared with you in the beginning of this chapter the Cruise Down Plate provides you the simplest method to support you in your goal of restoring your metabolism. There's no time-consuming calorie counting or banning of foods. As long as you fill the top half of your plate with veggies and the bottom half with equal portions of protein and carbohydrate foods along with 1 teaspoon of fat, you will provide your body the essential muscle-making materials to create new lean muscle – which will burn the fat!

some suggested guidelines

I've provided the following food lists to be used with your Jorge Cruise Planner on page 77 as an optional resource for those of you who want a little more security during your first week or two with the Cruise Down Plate. If you ever feel confused about how much food to place on your Cruise Down Plate, consult my simple food lists on the following pages.

Use these lists to measure out your food portions for 1 week. After that, you should be able to automatically judge your food portions without the need of measuring scales. Think of your first week as your week of training. Soon, you'll be ready to take off your training wheels and ride effortlessly on the road to weight loss!

approximate caloric values

Although I have done all the counting for you, just for your reference here are the approximate caloric values of all the boxes found on the Jorge Cruise Planner on page 77. All you need to do is check off the boxes on the planner and you are set!

Vegetable/Fruit	50
Fat	45
Carbohydrates	80
Protein	75
Snack	100
Treat	30–50

vegetables/fruits

vegetables

Vegetables that are high in starch do not appear on this list; they are on the Carbohydrates list. For each specified vegetable amount, check off 1 Veggie box on your planner. All servings are 230 g (8 oz) raw or 145 g (5 oz) cooked, unless otherwise stated:

- Artichoke, medium
- Asparagus
- Aubergine
- Beetroot
- Beetroot greens
- Broccoli
- Brussels sprouts
- Carrots
- Cauliflower
- Green beans
- Kale
- Leeks
- Mangetout
- Mung bean sprouts
- Onions
- Parsnips
- Peppers (green, yellow, red)
- Sauerkraut
- Seaweed, raw
- Sugar snap peas
- Swede
- Tomato (2 medium)
- Tomato purée (6 tablespoons)
- Tomatoes, canned (230 g/8 oz)
- Turnips
- Vegetable soup, fat-free, low sodium (240 ml/8 fl oz)

fruit

For each specified amount, check off 1 Fruit box on your Jorge Cruise Planner. If you can't find a particular fruit listed, check off 1 box for every small to medium fresh fruit, 125 g (4½ oz) of canned fruit, or 45 g (1½ oz) dried fruit. Ideally, eat fruit only for breakfast due to its higher simple sugar content.

- Apples, green or red (1 medium)
- Apple juice (120 ml/4 fl oz)
- Apple purée, unsweetened (120 ml/4 fl oz)
- Apricots (4)
- Bananas (½ medium)
- Blackberries (100 g/3½ oz)
- Blueberries (100 g/3½ oz)
- Cantaloupe (⅓ melon)
- Cherries (12 large)
- Cranberry juice (120 ml/4 fl oz)
- Fruit salad (125 g/4½ oz)
- Grapefruit (½)
- Grapefruit juice (120 ml/4 fl oz)
- Grapes, green or red (12)
- Honeydew (⅓ melon)
- Kiwi fruit (1 large)
- Orange (1 medium)
- Peach (1 medium)
- Pear (1 small)
- Pineapple, canned, packed in juice (125 g/4½ oz)
- Plums (2 medium)
- Prunes (2)
- Raisins (2 tablespoons)
- Raspberries (125 g/4½ oz)
- Strawberries (125 g/4½ oz)
- Watermelon (150 g/5½ oz)

fats

For each specified amount, cross off 1 Fat box on your Jorge Cruise Planner.

preferred fats

- Almond butter (1 tablespoon) PLUS 1 Protein box

- Almonds, raw (6)
- Avocado (⅛ medium)
- Cashews (6)
- Flax oil (1 teaspoon or 4 capsules)
- Oil-based salad dressing (1 tablespoon)
- Olive oil (1 teaspoon)
- Olives (10 small or 5 large)
- Peanut butter (2 teaspoons) PLUS 1 Protein box
- Peanuts (10)
- Pecans (4 halves)
- Pumpkin seeds (1 tablespoon)
- Sesame seeds (1 tablespoon)
- Soya mayonnaise (1 tablespoon)
- Sunflower seeds (1 tablespoon)
- Tahini paste (2 teaspoons)

fats to minimize

- Butter, reduced-calorie (1 tablespoon)
- Butter (1 teaspoon)
- Coconut (2 tablespoons)
- Cream cheese (1 tablespoon)
- Cream cheese, reduced-calorie (2 tablespoons)

- Mayonnaise (1 teaspoon)
- Mayonnaise, reduced-calorie (1 tablespoon)
- Single cream (2 tablespoons)
- Soured cream (2 tablespoons)
- Vegetable cooking fat (1 teaspoon)

carbohydrates

For each specified amount, check off 1 Carbohydrate box on your Jorge Cruise Planner. Higher-fat selections will require you to check off 1 or 2 Fat boxes in addition to the complex Carbohydrate box. If you can't find a particular complex carbohydrate listed, check off one box for every 60–90 g (2–3 oz) serving of cereal, grain, pasta, or starchy vegetable.

breads

- Bagel (½ of a 60-g/2-oz bagel)
- Bread (30 g/1 oz or 1 slice)
- English muffin (½)
- Hamburger bun (½)
- Naan bread (¼ of 20 x 5 cm/8 x 2 in loaf)
- Pitta, 15 cm/6 in (1/2)
- Roll, dinner (1 small)

- Tortilla, corn, 15 cm/6 in (1)
- Tortilla, flour, 18 cm/7 in (1)
- Waffle, fat-free (1)

cereals and grains

- Barley, cooked (90 g/3 oz)
- Basmati rice (60 g/2 oz)
- Brown rice, cooked (60 g/2 oz)
- Buckwheat (Kasha), cooked (90 g/3 oz)
- Bulgur wheat, cooked (90 g/3 oz)
- Cereal, cold, sweetened (20 g/¾ oz)
- Cereal, cold, unsweetened (30 g/1 oz)
- Cereal, hot (90 g/3 oz)
- Couscous, cooked (90 g/3 oz)
- Muesli, unsweetened (30 g/1 oz)
- Wheat germ (3 tablespoons)
- Wild rice, cooked (50 g/1½ oz)

flour

- Cornflour (2 tablespoons)
- Matzo meal (5 tablespoons)
- Wholemeal flour (2½ tablespoons)

pasta

- All varieties cooked such as spaghetti, linguine, noodles, penne (75 g/2½ oz)

starchy vegetables

- Corn (75 g/2½ oz)
- Corn on the cob (15-cm/6-in ear)
- French fries (10) PLUS 1 Fat box
- Green peas (75 g/2½ oz)
- Potato, baked (1 small)
- Potato, instant (75 g/2½ oz)
- Potato, mashed (115 g/4 oz)
- Pumpkin (125 g/4½ oz)
- Sweet potato (115 g/4 oz)
- Winter squash, acorn or butternut (185 g/6½ oz)

crackers

- Matzo (20 g/¾ oz)
- Melba toast (4 slices)
- Wholewheat crackers (2–5)

protein

For each specified amount, check off 1 Protein box on your Jorge Cruise Planner. Higher-fat selections will require you to check off 1 or 2 Fat boxes in addition to the Protein box. Meat protein sources are based on cooked portions; raw meat will shrink when cooking. A 115 g (4 oz) raw chicken breast will shrink to 90 g (3 oz) when cooked.

beans

- Black, cooked (90 g/3 oz)
- Chickpeas, cooked (90 g/3 oz)
- Hummus (4 level tablespoons) PLUS 1 Fat box
- Kidney, cooked (90 g/3 oz)
- Lentil, cooked (90 g/3 oz)
- Lima, cooked (90 g/3 oz)
- Pinto, cooked (90 g/3 oz)
- Refried, fat-added (90 g/3 oz) PLUS 1 Fat box
- Split peas, cooked (90 g/3 oz)
- White, cooked (90 g/3 oz)

cheese

- Boursin light (60 g/2 oz)
- Brie, half-fat (40 g/1½ oz)
- Cheddar, half-fat (30 g/1 oz)
- Cottage cheese, natural (60 g/2 oz)
- Feta (30 g/1 oz)
- Goat's (30 g/1 oz)
- Mozzarella (30 g/1 oz)
- Parmesan, freshly grated (20 g/¾ oz)
- Ricotta (60 g/2 oz)
- Swiss (20 g/¾ oz)

milk products

- Lactose-free milk, low-fat or fat-free (180 ml/6 fl oz)
- Milk, skimmed (180 ml/6 fl oz)
- Skimmed dry milk (5 tablespoons)
- Soya milk, fortified, skimmed (180 ml/6 fl oz)
- Yogurt, frozen, low-fat or fat-free (2 scoops)
- Yogurt, low-fat or fat-free, flavoured (170 g/6 oz) PLUS check off 2 Fruit boxes
- Yogurt, low-fat or fat-free, plain (170 g/6 oz)

eggs

- Egg, whole (1)
- Egg substitute (4 tablespoons)

- Egg whites (3)

poultry

- Chicken or turkey, white meat without skin (30 g/1 oz)

- Chicken or turkey, dark meat with skin (30 g/1 oz)

fish, canned

- Salmon, packed in water (60 g/2 oz)

- Sardines, packed in water (2 medium)

- Tuna, packed in water (60 g/2 oz)

fish, fresh or frozen

- Fried fish (30 g/1 oz) PLUS 1 Fat box

- Salmon (30 g/1 oz)

- Sea bass (30 g/1 oz)

- Sole (30 g/1 oz)

- Swordfish (30 g/1 oz)

- Tuna (30 g/1 oz)

shellfish

- Clams (60 g/2 oz)

- Crab (60 g/2 oz)

- Crayfish (60 g/2 oz)

- Lobster (60 g/2 oz)

- Oysters (6 medium)

- Prawns (60 g/2 oz)

- Scallops (60 g/2 oz)

soya products

- Soya beans, cooked (90 g/3 oz)

- Soya burger (½ burger)

- Soya cheese (30 g/1 oz)

- Soya hot dog (1)

- Soya milk, fortified, skimmed (180 ml/6 fl oz)

- Texturized soya protein (2 tablespoons)

- Tofu (90 g/3 oz)

red meats

- Bacon (1 rasher) PLUS 1 Fat box

- Ham, smoked or fresh (30 g/1 oz)

- Hot dog, beef or pork (1) PLUS 2 Fat boxes

- Lamb shank or shoulder (30 g/1 oz)

- Pork fillet (30 g/1 oz)

- Sirloin steak (30 g/1 oz)

- Stewing steak (30 g/1 oz)

- Topside (30 g/1 oz)

- Veal chop or roast (30 g/1 oz)

- Venison (30 g/1 oz)

snacks

For each specified amount, check off 1 snack box on your Jorge Cruise Planner. In general, your snacks are about 100 calories.

- Almonds (12)

- Angel food cake (60 g/2 oz)

- Baby carrots (230 g/8 oz)

- Brownie (5-cm/2-in square)

- Butterscotch (4 pieces)

- Cadbury's Heroes (2)

- Cashews (12)

- Celery (3 sticks with 1 teaspoon of peanut butter on each)

- Cereal bar, low-fat (1)

- Chocolate-covered almonds (7)

- Dime bar (½)

- Fruit, 1 piece (see fruit lists for portion size)

- Fudge (30 g/1 oz)

- Kit Kat (1 2-piece bar)

- Melba toast (4 slices)

- Peanut brittle (30 g/1 oz)

- Peanuts (20)

- Pecans (8 halves)

- Popcorn, air popped (2 handfuls)

- Potato crisps, low-fat (23-g/¾-oz bag)

- Pretzels (20 g/¾ oz)

- Pumpkin seeds (2 tablespoons)

- Raisins (30)

- Rice cakes (2 small)

- Sesame seeds (2 tablespoons)

- Sorbet (2 scoops)

- String cheese (1)

- Sunflower seeds (2 tablespoons)

- Tortilla chips, low-fat (8–10)

- Wholewheat crackers (2–5)

- Yogurt, frozen, low-fat or fat-free (75 g/2½ oz)

- Yogurt, low-fat or fat-free (230 g/8 oz)

treats

For each specified amount, check off 1 treat box on your Jorge Cruise Planner. Eat a delicious treat every day. In general, they should be 30 to 50 calories.

- Biscuit (1 small)

- Boiled sweets (1)

- Cheese slice, reduced-calorie (1)

- Chocolate chips (½ tablespoon)

- Chocolate-coated mints (2)

- Cookie, fat-free (1 small)

- Frozen seedless grapes (115 g/4 oz)

- Fruit gums (3–4 small)

- Jelly beans (7)

- Licorice sweet (1)

- Marshmallow (1 large)

- M&M's (¼ of small bag)

- Popcorn, air popped (1 handful)

- Sorbet (1 scoop)

alcohol

For maximum weight loss, alcohol should be kept to a minimum and limited to special occasions. Check off 1 snack box on your Jorge Cruise Planner for each of the specified amounts.

- Beer (350 ml/12 fl oz)

- Spirits (30 ml/1 fl oz)

- Wine (150 ml/5 fl oz)

freebies

The following items do not need to be counted and you can consume them as often as you like. These are great items to use if you want a second plate of food or more than your two daily snacks. Enjoy them!

vegetables

- Alfalfa sprouts

- Cabbage

- Celery

- Chilli peppers

- Courgettes

- Cucumber

- Garlic

- Lettuce, all types (iceberg, loose leaf, romaine, spinach, watercress)

- Mushrooms

- Onions

- Radishes

- Spring onions

drinks

- Carbonated or mineral water (add lime or lemon for great taste!)

- Coffee, plain

- Soft drinks, calorie-free

- Tea

Note: For each beverage you drink that contains caffeine you must increase your water intake by 2 extra glasses to stay hydrated.

seasonings

- Garlic

- Herbs, fresh or dried

- Non-stick olive oil cooking spray

- Salsas, Tabasco, Worcestershire sauce or hot pepper sauce

- Spices

condiments

- Horseradish

- Lemon juice

- Lime juice

- Mustard

- Soy sauce, light

- Vinegar

sugar substitutes

- Equal

- Splenda

- Sweet and Low

miscellaneous

- Sugar-free chewing gum

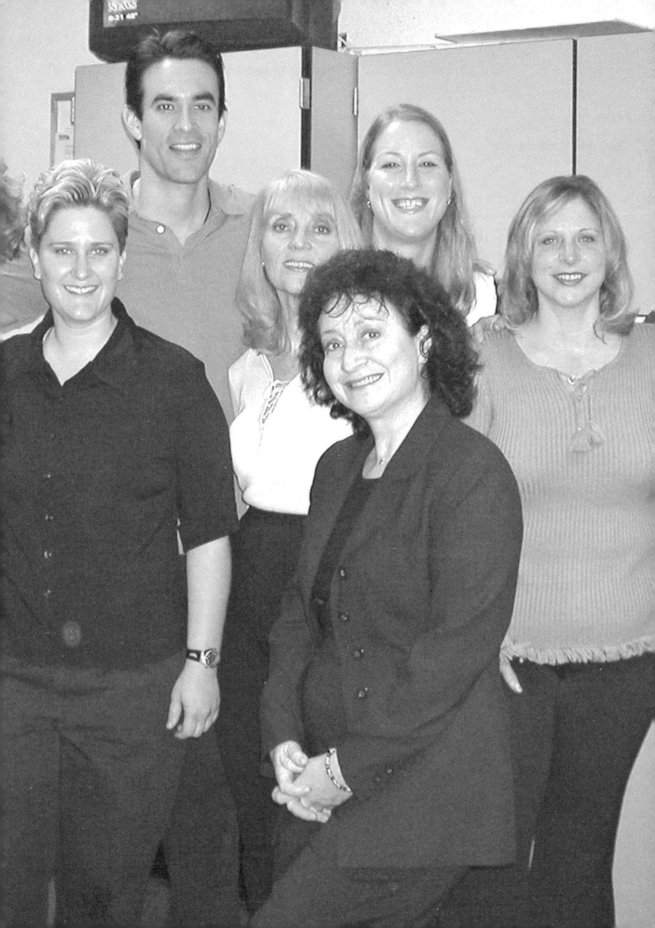

Part 3
The Programme

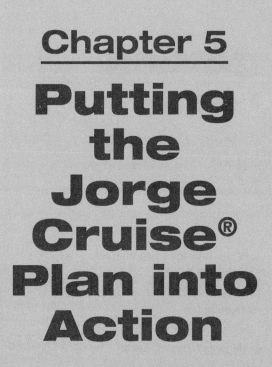

Chapter 5

Putting the Jorge Cruise® Plan into Action

Use This 3-Level Plan to Slim Your Hips and Thighs

getting ready

Welcome to your *8 Minutes in the Morning for Lean Hips and Thin Thighs* programme. This is where the rubber meets the road, so to speak, because you will be putting everything you've just learned into action.

In the following pages you'll find three different programmes, ranging in difficulty from gentle to challenging.

Start with Level 1, the gentlest of the programmes. Each programme starts on a Monday and ends on a Sunday. You'll repeat each programme for 3 weeks before moving onto the next level. In other words, you'll start Level 1 on a Monday and follow it for 21 days, starting over each Monday. After 21 days, you'll advance to Level 2. After 21 more days, you'll advance to Level 3.

If you are already fairly fit, Level 1 may feel too easy for you. If you don't feel challenged by the exercises, you may move up to Level 2 after just one week.

your '8 minute' edge

During each week of your *8 Minutes in the Morning for Lean Hips and Thin Thighs* journey, you will:

• Feel your hips and thighs become tighter, firmer and stronger

• Lose up to 1 kg (2 lb) of fat a week

• Create long, lean, sexy legs

using the programme

Each day during your Monday through Friday sessions, you will find a power thought to help keep you motivated, four Cruise Moves and a visualization that will help you to eat nutritionally and not emotionally.

Always start your morning with your Cruise Moves – they are the core of the programme and your most important ally in slimming your hips and thighs. Your sessions Monday, Wednesday and Friday will focus on your trouble zone – your hips and thighs. Your Tuesday sessions will focus on your upper body and your Thursday sessions will target your midsection and calves.

Warm up by jogging on the spot for 1 minute. Then do each Cruise Move for 1 minute and move on to the next Cruise Move. After you've completed all four moves, repeat each move one time for a total of 8 minutes. Then cool down with the stretches suggested on page 74.

Each day of the programme you will find a powerful visualization to help you overcome emotional eating and stay motivated. When you create an image in your mind of what you want to accomplish, you take the first crucial step to making your dreams a reality. The visualizations in this programme will help you more effectively deal with negative emotions that may have caused you to overeat in the past,

a 2-step format

Each day of the programme follows a simple format. Each day you do two things:

Step 1.
8 Minutes Moves®
(Cruise Moves)

Step 2.
Eat Nutritionally, *Not* Emotionally®

confront difficult people and situations that sometimes trigger mood swings, and build a strong internal motivation to follow a healthy diet.

During your visualizations, you need to draw on all of your senses: touch, taste, smell, sight and sound. The more senses you involve in your visualizations, the more powerful your images will become and the more effective your time spent.

how weekends work

You will tackle your weekends a little differently than your Monday through Friday sessions. You'll take each weekend off from your Cruise Moves, but not from building lean muscle and taking additional steps toward your goal. Each Saturday you will find four stretches for the hip and thigh zone. These stretches will help *elongate* your muscles. They are an optional component of the programme. However, they take only 8 minutes, and they will greatly *accelerate* your results. (You'll find additional optional ways to accelerate your results in the bonus chapter on page 199.)

Each Sunday you will also take the day off from Cruise Moves. However, take a moment to capture your progress by weighing yourself and taking your hip and thigh measurements. Also, feel free to enjoy your stronger body by taking a hike, playing a game with your kids, or going for a walk in the park.

your homework

Before you get started on your new adventure, you'll need to make sure you have the tools for the journey. Please don't start the programme until you:

1. Purchase your equipment. You need minimal equipment for *8 Minutes in the Morning for Lean Hips and Thin Thighs*. When you get to Level 3, I suggest you try the hips and legs exercises with a pair of ankle weights, available at most good sports stores. These small weights easily strap to your ankles and will help add resistance, making your Cruise Moves more effective.

2. Read chapters 1 through 4. Please don't start the programme without first reading about how it works and understanding the formula behind the 2-step process.

3. Write down your current weight and measurements and take a 'before' photo. Your original weight, hips and thighs circumference, and before photo will not only help serve as powerful reminders of your goal, but they will also help you to see your progress. To take your measurements, use a flexible tape measure. Wrap it around your hips at their widest point. Then do the same with your thighs, wrapping it around your thigh roughly mid-distance between your knee and hipbone. Record your measurements and weight in the space provided on the opposite page.

4. Determine your goal. Sure, you want leaner hips and thinner thighs, but how much leaner? How many kilos down? I recommend you pick a goal weight. That way you'll know when you've reached your goal! To pick a goal weight, consult the height and weight chart on the opposite page. Find your age on the chart and match that to your height. There you will find a healthy weight range for someone your age and size. Use that to determine your goal. Write your goal in the space provided.

You also might want to choose a motivational goal as well, one that is not tied to the scale. For example, do you have a pair of jeans that you can no longer wear? You might want to write that down as a goal, too.

5. Determine how long it will take to reach your goal. You'll find out how to do just that by consulting the chart on the opposite page.

your cooldown stretches

After your Cruise Moves, do the following stretches to cool down and increase your flexibility.

Sky-reaching pose. Stand tall and reach with both hands toward the sky as high as you comfortably can. Feel the stretch lengthening your spine, bringing more range of motion to your joints. Breathe deeply through your nose. Hold from 10 seconds to 1 minute.

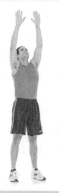

Cobra stretch. Lie on a towel or mat on your belly with your palms flat on the ground next to your shoulders and your legs just slightly less than shoulder-width apart. Your feet should be resting on their tops. Lift your upper body up off the ground, inhaling through

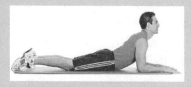

your nose as you rise. Press your hips into the floor and curve your upper body backward, looking up. This stretch is one that you may need to work up to, so right now, do the best you can. Hold from 10 seconds to 1 minute.

Hurdler's stretch. Sit on a towel or mat on the floor with your legs extended in front of you. Keeping your back straight, gently bend forward from the hips and reach as far as you can toward your toes. If possible, pull your toes back slightly toward your upper body. Again, don't worry if this stretch is difficult for you right now – do the best you can. Eventually, you'll get it! Hold from 10 seconds to 1 minute.

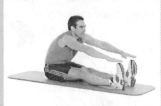

your current body
and future goals

To find your healthy weight, find your age and height on the chart below. You know yourself better than anyone else does, so select a number that is realistic for you. Subtract that number from your current weight. That's your weight-loss goal.

Then, to determine a target date for achieving this goal, divide your goal weight by two. That's the number of weeks it will take to reach your goal. Consult a calendar and find the date you will achieve your goal weight, then record your answers to the following:

1. What is your current weight? _____

2. What is your current thigh circumference? _____

3. What is your current hip circumference? _____

your future body

1. What is your goal weight? _____

2. How many weeks will it take to reach your goal weight? _____

3. What is your goal thigh circumference? _____

4. What is your goal hip circumference? _____

5. List any other goals: _____

your weight chart

Height	Weight (lb/kg)		Height	Weight (lb/kg)	
	19–34 yr	*35+ yr*		*19–34 yr*	*35+ yr*
5'0" (1.52 m)	6 st 13 lb–9 st 2 lb (44–58 kg)	7 st 10 lb–9 st 12 lb (49–63 kg)	5'8" (1.72 m)	8 st 13 lb–11 st 10 lb (57–75 kg)	9 st 12 lb–12 st 10 lb (63–81 kg)
5'1" (1.54 m)	7 st 3 lb–9 st 6 lb (46–60 kg)	7 st 13 lb–10 st 3 lb (50–65 kg)	5'9" (1.75 m)	9 st 3 lb–12 st 1 lb (59–77 kg)	10 st 2 lb–13 st 1 lb (65–83 kg)
5'2" (1.57 m)	7 st 6 lb–9 st 11 lb (47–62 kg)	8 st 3 lb–10 st 8 lb (52–67 kg)	5'10" (1.77 m)	9 st 6 lb–12 st 6 lb (60–79 kg)	10 st 6 lb–13 st 6 lb (66–85 kg)
5'3" (1.60 m)	7 st 9 lb–10 st 1 lb (49–64 kg)	8 st 7 lb–10 st 12 lb (54–69 kg)	5'11" (1.80 m)	9 st 10 lb–12 st 11 lb (62–81 kg)	10 st 11 lb–13 st 12 lb (69–88 kg)
5'4" (1.62 m)	7 st 13 lb–10 st 6 lb (50–66 kg)	8 st 10 lb–11 st 13 lb (55–71 kg)	6'0" (1.83 m)	10 st–13 st 2 lb (64–84 kg)	11 st 1 lb–14 st 3 lb (70–90 kg)
5'5" (1.65 m)	8 st 2 lb–10 st 10 lb (52–68 kg)	9 st–11 st 8 lb (57–74 kg)	6'1" (1.85 m)	10 st 4 lb–13 st 7 lb (65–86 kg)	11 st 5 lb–14 st 9 lb (72–93 kg)
5'6" (1.67 m)	8 st 6 lb–11 st 1 lb (54–70 kg)	9 st 4 lb–11 st 13 lb (59–76 kg)	6'2" (1.88 m)	10 st 8 lb–13 st 13 lb (67–89 kg)	11 st 10 lb–15st (75–95 kg)
5'7" (1.70 m)	8 st 9 lb–11 st 6 lb (55–73 kg)	9 st 8 lb–12 st 4 lb (61–78 kg)	6'3" (1.91 m)	10 st 12 lb–14st 4lb (69–91 kg)	12st–15st 6lb (76–98 kg)

SOURCE: U.S. Department of Health and Human Services, Dietary Guidelines for Americans

MY 'BEFORE' AND 'AFTER' PHOTOS

Your 'before' and 'after' photos will help motivate you to stay focused on your weight-loss goal.
Review this page each day to *prevent* emotional eating. Take your 'before' photo
right now and paste them on this page. But don't wait to see your future body!
You can go to www.myvirtualmodel.com and print out your 'after' photo right now.
Photocopy this page for each day of the programme and use it to keep yourself organized.

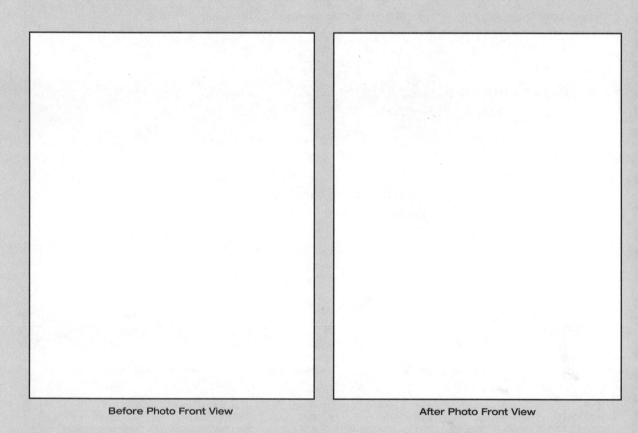

Before Photo Front View   After Photo Front View

Instructions for using the planner: Make seven copies for each week. Then, stack them and staple in the upper left-hand corner. Keep them with you at all times.

JORGE CRUISE®
LEAN HIP & THIN THIGH PLANNER

Date _____

Step 1: 8 Minutes Moves®

Muscle-Making Routine:
Monday: Hips and Thighs Day
Tuesday: Upper Body
Wednesday: Hips and Thighs Day
Thursday: Lower Body
Friday: Hips and Thighs Day
Saturday: Stretch Day
Sunday: Day Off

	Set 1	Set 2
Move 1:		
Move 2:		
Move 3:		
Move 4:		

In each 'Move' box, write down the Cruise Move® and then in the 'Set 1 and Set 2' box, keep track of the number of reps performed or time held.

Step 2: Eat Nutritionally, Not Emotionally®

Muscle-Making Material:
Veggies: Salad, Steamed Veggies, or 1 Fruit
Fat: 1 tsp of Flax, Olive Oil, or Butter
Carbs: 60–90 g (2–3 oz) of a grain or 1 slice of bread
Protein: 30 g (1 oz) of Fish/Chicken/Meat/Cheese, 3 Egg Whites, 90 g (3 oz) of Beans, or 1 Glass of Skimmed Milk
Snacks: 100-calorie Item
Treat: 30- to 50-calorie Item

Each box equals an above example. Eat every 3 hours and stop eating 3 hours before bed.

Water (✔): 8 fl oz Glass

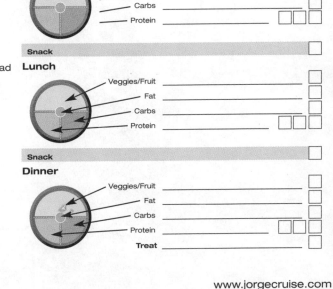

Breakfast
Veggies/Fruit _____
Fat _____
Carbs _____
Protein _____

Snack

Lunch
Veggies/Fruit _____
Fat _____
Carbs _____
Protein _____

Snack

Dinner
Veggies/Fruit _____
Fat _____
Carbs _____
Protein _____
Treat _____

www.jorgecruise.com

77

Level 1
Monday

'One can never
consent to creep
when one feels an
impulse to soar.'

Helen Keller

jorge's power thought

Today you take an important step forward toward your goal of leaner hips and thinner thighs. I want you to congratulate yourself for getting this far. Often getting started is half the battle. The other half of the battle? Sticking with it.

You may know from personal experience that losing weight and slimming down is only part of the effort. Staying that way and preventing weight gain is the other part. The way to keep the weight off? Make a commitment today that you will stick with this programme for good! *8 Minutes in the Morning for Lean Hips and Thin Thighs* is not a temporary fix for your body. Rather, it's a lifestyle. So stop thinking thoughts such as, 'I only need to keep this up for 4 weeks'. You must maintain it for life!

And here's some great news. The *8 Minutes in the Morning for Lean Hips and Thin Thighs* programme is the easiest programme to keep up. My clients often tell me how it has become an integral part of their lives. No programme is easier and more convenient. So make the commitment now, on day 1 of your journey, to make that lifestyle change and become a Jorge Cruise® client for life!

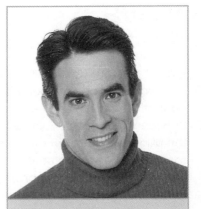

'You only need 8 minutes a day to slim down and stay that way. It's the most effective 8 minutes you can ever spend on your body.'

8 minute moves®
thighs day

MOVE 1: seated pillow squeeze
inner thighs

a. Sit on a sturdy chair (one without wheels). Rest your feet on the floor with your knees bent at 90-degree angles. Place a pillow between your thighs. Exhale as you squeeze the pillow between your thighs, as if you were trying to squeeze the stuffing out of the pillow. Hold for 1 minute as you breathe normally. Release and proceed to Move 2.

a

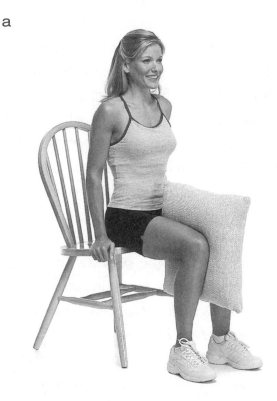

8-MINUTE LOG				
exercise	move 1	move 2	move 3	move 4
sets				
reps				

MOVE 2: seated hand push
outer thighs and hips

a. Sit on a sturdy chair. Rest your feet on the floor with your knees bent at 90-degree angles. Place your palms on the outsides of your knees. While keeping your palms and arms stationary, push your knees outward against your palms, as if you were trying to push your palms away. At the same time, press inward with your hands, preventing your thighs from pushing them outward. Hold this isometric contraction for 1 minute, breathing normally. Release and proceed to Move 3 on page 82.

a

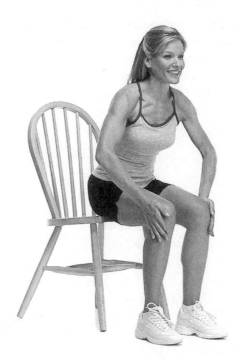

exercise sequence

1. warm up Jog or march on the spot for 1 minute.

2. cruise moves Do one 60-second repetition of each of your 4 Cruise Moves. Repeat this cycle and you will be done in 8 minutes.

3. cool down After your Cruise Moves, do these stretches (see page 74).

Sky-reaching pose | Hurdler's stretch | Cobra stretch

thighs day (cont'd)

MOVE 3: seated leg raise
fronts of the thighs

a. Sit on a sturdy chair. Rest your feet on the floor with your knees bent at 90-degree angles. Rest your hands on the chair at your sides. Exhale as you lift and extend your right leg. Hold for 30 seconds as you breathe normally. Then inhale as you lower your right leg and exhale as you repeat with your left leg. Hold for 30 seconds while breathing normally. Release and proceed to Move 4.

a

eat nutritionally, *not* emotionally®
visualization

To help make sure you eat nutritionally and not emotionally, you can use a powerful mind-body technique called vivid visualization to help you stay emotionally strong and empowered. Today's visualization will help you fill up the void in your heart that may be leading to overeating. To begin, close your eyes and take a few deep, relaxing breaths in through your nose, out through your mouth. Allow each exhalation to bring you to a state of deep relaxation. Once you feel completely relaxed, you're ready to begin.

MOVE 4: seated bridge
backs of the thighs and rear end

a. Sit on the edge of a sturdy chair. Rest your feet on the floor with your knees bent at 90-degree angles. Rest your palms on the chair at your sides. Exhale as you lift your hips, allowing your palms and feet to support your body weight. Continue to lift your hips until your body resembles the shape of a bridge. Hold for 20 to 60 seconds while breathing normally. Release and return to Move 1 on page 80. Repeat Moves 1–4 once more, and you're done.

a

filling your void

Imagine a group of loving and compassionate people – ones you know in real life, or religious and historical figures – gathered with you. Imagine that they merge together to form a sphere of bright, warm, healing energy. See this energy move into your heart, filling it with love. Now, imagine that your heart glows and radiates love and that this radiating, warm light fills up every space so that your heart feels warm, full and content.

Allow this loving energy to transcend the confines of your heart and fill up your entire body. As it fills up every nook and cranny, feel any negativity – anger, sadness, fear – become squeezed out of your body. Feel yourself grow happy, joyful and content.

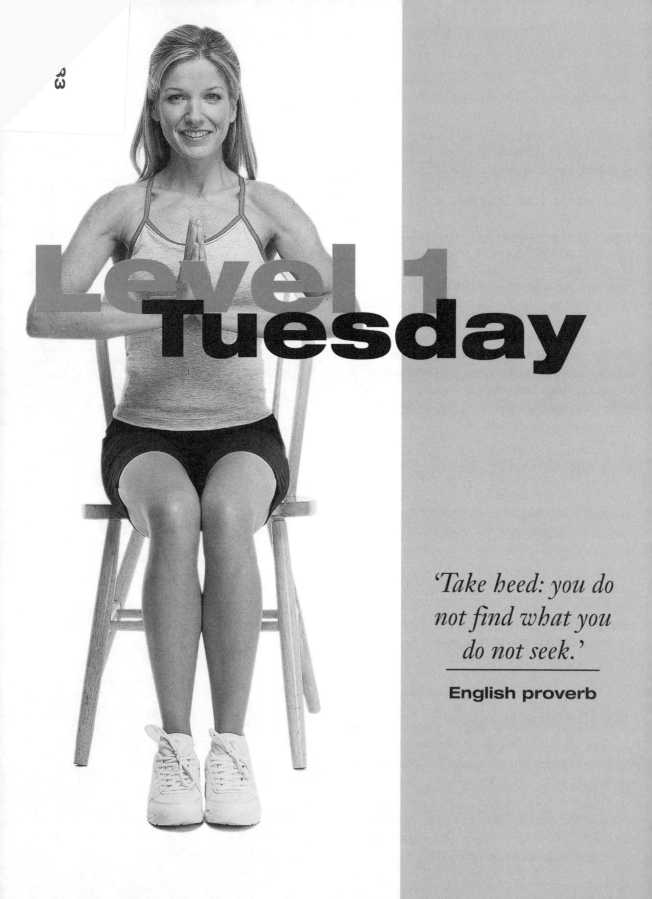

Level 1
Tuesday

'Take heed: you do
not find what you
do not seek.'

English proverb

jorge's power thought

Don't feel tempted to skip your Cruise Moves today. I know the reasoning. You might be thinking, 'My true trouble zone is my thighs. I targeted them yesterday, so I might as well take today off'. Don't let such thoughts talk you into hitting the snooze button on your alarm clock! Believe me, your 8 minutes in the morning today are better spent doing your Cruise Moves than sleeping!

As I've mentioned before, you must create muscle all over your body – including your arms, shoulders, chest and back – to see true, lasting results. It's the muscle that you create all over your body that helps boost your metabolism high enough to burn the excess fat in your hips and thighs. If you target only your trouble zone, you won't slim your thighs. Also, your Cruise Moves for the upper body will help lift your breasts (if you're a woman) and firm underarm flab, a trouble spot for most people. Today's moves will help you shape strong, sexy arms and shoulders. They are crucial to your success.

So promise me right now that you will treat your non–trouble zone Cruise Moves today with the respect they deserve. Again, it's the best 8 minutes you will ever spend on your body. So get out of bed and get moving!

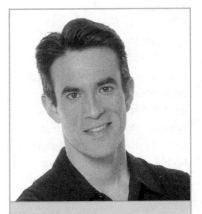

'Accept and nurture your body. Only then will nutrition and exercise efforts become effortless.'

8 minute moves®
upper-body day

MOVE 1: squeeze hold
chest

a. Sit in a sturdy chair (one without wheels) with your feet flat on the floor. Bend your arms and exhale as you press the palms of your hands together at chest level. Once in position, keep your chest tight and flexed. Hold firmly for 60 seconds as you breathe normally, then proceed to Move 2.

a

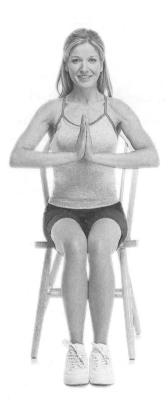

8-MINUTE LOG				
exercise	move 1	move 2	move 3	move 4
sets				
reps				

MOVE 2: pull down hold
upper back

a. Sit 60–90 cm (2–3 ft) in front of a table on a sturdy chair with your feet flat on the floor. Bend forward from your hips and extend your arms onto the top of the table, placing your palms against the tabletop. Exhale as you press down onto the table. Hold firmly for 60 seconds as you breathe normally, then proceed to Move 3 on page 88.

a

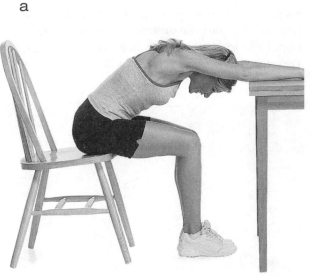

exercise sequence

1. warm up Jog or march on the spot for 1 minute.

2. cruise moves Do one 60-second repetition of each of your 4 Cruise Moves. Repeat this cycle and you will be done in 8 minutes.

3. cool down After your Cruise Moves, do these stretches (see page 74).

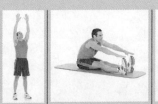

Sky-reaching pose | Hurdler's stretch | Cobra stretch

upper-body day (cont'd)

MOVE 3: push down hold
biceps

a. Sit about 60 cm (2 ft) away from a table in a sturdy chair with your feet flat on the floor. Place your palms on the table with your elbows bent about 90 degrees. Exhale as you press down into the tabletop as hard as you can. Hold for 60 seconds, breathing normally. Release and proceed to Move 4.

a

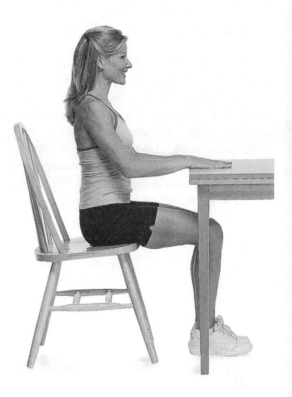

eat nutritionally, *not* emotionally®
visualization

Today you will continue to nurture your heart with another visualization exercise, helping to fill up any void that may lead to overeating. Close your eyes and take a few deep, relaxing breaths, in through your nose and out through your mouth. Feel your body relax more every time you exhale. Once you feel completely relaxed, you're ready to start.

MOVE 4: lift hold
triceps

a. Sit about 60 cm (2 ft) away from a table in a sturdy chair with your feet flat on the floor. Place your palms under the tabletop with your elbows bent about 90 degrees. Push up on the underside of the table as hard as you can. Hold firmly for 60 seconds, breathing normally. Release and return to Move 1 on page 86. Repeat Moves 1–4 once more and you're done.

a

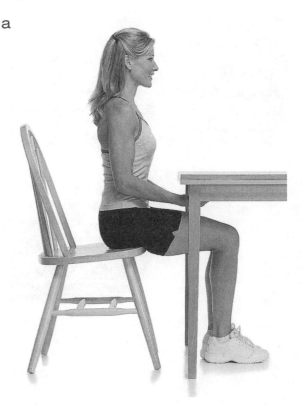

unconditional love

Imagine someone who loves you or loved you very deeply in the past (it's okay if you choose someone who has passed away). You might think of a parent or spouse or sibling or good friend. This person loves you unconditionally. Notice every feature of his or her face. Recall a time when this person displayed an act of unconditional love toward you.

Recall every detail of this memory. Remember how it felt to let someone love and nurture you. Allow your heart to feel grateful for this loving memory.

Now explore how your heart feels. Did the love from this person help to fill up your heart? Allow your heart to open up and enjoy the love that you've just created.

Level 1
Wednesday

'There are no
shortcuts to any
place worth going.'

Unknown

jorge's power thought

From working with millions of online clients, I've learned that you must first accept your body – with all of its quirks and inconveniences – before you can change your body. I've also learned that people who want to improve their hip and thigh zone often most need this advice.

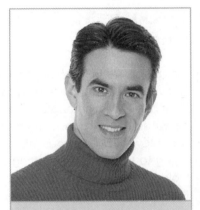

Take a moment to reflect upon your feelings about your body. How do you feel about your hips and thighs? Often when I ask my clients this question, a whole slew of negative thoughts pop up for them. Such nasty thoughts can unravel your best intentions. They erode your self-confidence and motivation to succeed. That's why you must get past those thoughts to experience true, lasting results.

How do you get past thinking negatively about your body shape? One of my clients developed what I now call the 'Oops' technique. Whenever you find yourself thinking something like, 'My thighs are hideous' or 'Even an elephant has slimmer legs than me', just say 'Oops' out loud. It may sound silly, but it helps to remind you to stop such negative thoughts and return your thinking to the positive. Remember, your hips and thighs are a precious gift. They allow you to walk! What would you do without them?

'If you don't fully accept your body, you will never treat it as the most precious gift that has ever been given to you.'

8 minute moves®
thighs day

MOVE 1: seated pillow squeeze
inner thighs

a. Sit on a sturdy chair (one without wheels).
Rest your feet on the floor with your knees
bent at 90-degree angles. Place a pillow
between your thighs. Exhale as you squeeze
the pillow between your thighs, as if you were
trying to squeeze the stuffing out of the pillow.
Hold for 1 minute as you breathe normally.
Release and proceed to Move 2.

a

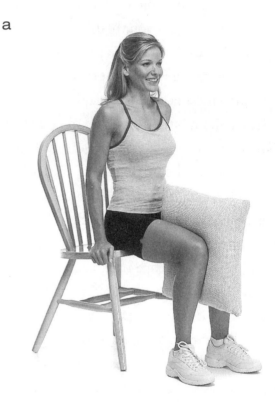

8-MINUTE LOG				
exercise	move 1	move 2	move 3	move 4
sets				
reps				

MOVE 2: seated hand push
outer thighs and hips

a. Sit on a sturdy chair. Rest your feet on the floor with your knees bent at 90-degree angles. Place your palms on the outsides of your knees. While keeping your palms and arms stationary, push your knees outward against your palms, as if you were trying to push your palms away. At the same time, press inward with your hands, preventing your thighs from pushing them outward. Hold this isometric contraction for 1 minute, breathing normally. Release and proceed to Move 3 on page 94.

a

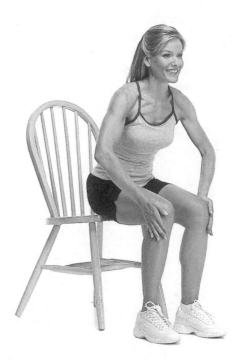

exercise sequence

1. warm up Jog or march on the spot for 1 minute.

2. cruise moves Do one 60-second repetition of each of your 4 Cruise Moves. Repeat this cycle and you will be done in 8 minutes.

3. cool down After your Cruise Moves, do these stretches (see page 74).

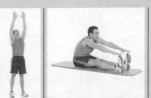
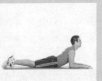

Sky-reaching pose | Hurdler's stretch | Cobra stretch

thighs day (cont'd)

MOVE 3: seated leg raise
fronts of the thighs

a. Sit on a sturdy chair. Rest your feet on the floor with your knees bent at 90-degree angles. Rest your hands on the chair at your sides. Exhale as you lift and extend your right leg. Hold for 30 seconds as you breathe normally. Then inhale as you lower your right leg and exhale as you repeat with your left leg. Hold for 30 seconds while breathing normally. Release and proceed to Move 4.

a

eat nutritionally, *not* emotionally®
visualization

Today you will again fill up your heart with love. You will expand on the visualization that you learned yesterday. Close your eyes and take a few deep, relaxing breaths, in through your nose and out through your mouth. Allow each exhalation to relax you more and more deeply. Once you feel completely relaxed, you are ready to begin.

MOVE 4: seated bridge
backs of the thighs and rear end

a. Sit on the edge of a sturdy chair. Rest your feet on the floor with your knees bent at 90-degree angles. Rest your palms on the chair at your sides. Exhale as you lift your hips, allowing your palms and feet to support your body weight. Continue to lift your hips until your body resembles the shape of a bridge. Hold for 20 to 60 seconds while breathing normally. Release and return to Move 1 on page 92. Repeat Moves 1–4 once more and you're done.

a

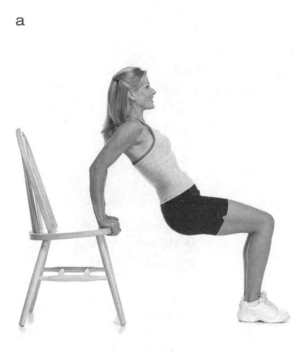

extend your love

Imagine someone who loves you or has loved you very deeply. It may be the same person you imagined yesterday, or it may be someone new. Recall a specific instance when this person displayed unconditional love for you and allow your heart to be open to receiving this love – even if it wasn't open in real life. Feel your heart fill up and then overflow with gratitude and love.

Now, imagine that you are sending some love back to this loved one. Feel as if the two of you are joined by a continuously circulating current of loving feelings. See this person smile and glow with the warmth of the love you have shared. Feel good about yourself for sharing the love you have created with someone else.

Level 1
Thursday

'They always say
time changes
things, but you
actually have to
change them
yourself.'

Andy Warhol

jorge's power thought

I've heard just about all of the excuses that were ever invented for not exercising or following a healthy diet. You know what? They are all lies. For example, here's one I hear all the time: people tell me that they don't have time to exercise. Not true. You need only 8 minutes a day. Who doesn't have 8 minutes?

Here's another one. I hear people make comments like, 'Weight loss is not worth the effort. I'm just going to gain it back.' You'll gain it back only if you stop practising your new health habits. As long as you continue to stick to your Cruise Moves and Cruise Down Plate, any weight you lose will stay off.

Most of the lies that we tell ourselves stem from one giant lie. That lie is this: 'I'm not good enough'. When you believe you're not good enough, then you believe that you don't have the time to put into it. When you believe you're not good enough, you fail to make exercise and healthy eating a priority. The visualizations that you complete throughout your journey to lean hips and thin thighs will help you see that. For now, however, I want you to replace that lie with the truth. The truth is that **you *are* worth it**. The truth is that your current body is the most precious gift you have ever been given.

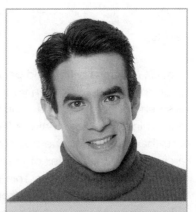

'I know from my most successful clients that real weight loss happens only when your body becomes your highest priority.'

8 minute moves®
torso and calves day

MOVE 1: stir hold
belly

a. Sit or stand with good posture. Lengthen your spine and straighten your back. Relax your shoulders. Exhale as you tighten your abdominal muscles. Make a fist with one of your hands and rub the bottom of your fist in a circle over the center of your navel as if you were stirring cake batter. This will force you to keep your abs contracted strongly. Hold for 60 seconds as you breathe normally. Release and proceed to Move 2.

a

8-MINUTE LOG				
exercise	move 1	move 2	move 3	move 4
sets				
reps				

MOVE 2: superman hold
lower back

a. Stand in front of a sturdy chair (one without wheels) with your left foot directly under your left hip. Bend forward and place your left palm on the chair seat, just under your left shoulder. Exhale as you raise and extend your right leg back and your right arm forward, forming a straight line from foot to fingertips. Hold for 30 seconds, release, and repeat on the other side. Then proceed to Move 3 on page 100.

a

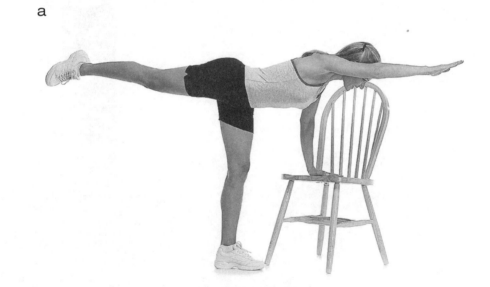

exercise sequence

1. warm up Jog or march on the spot for 1 minute.

2. cruise moves Do one 60-second repetition of each of your 4 Cruise Moves. Repeat this cycle and you will be done in 8 minutes.

3. cool down After your Cruise Moves, do these stretches (see page 74).

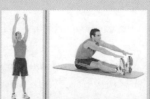
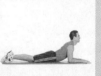

Sky-reaching pose | **Hurdler's stretch** | **Cobra stretch**

torso and calves day (cont'd)

MOVE 3: airplane hold
shoulders

a. Sit or stand. Exhale and raise your arms out to your sides. Stop once your arms reach shoulder height. Keep your shoulders relaxed away from your ears. Hold firmly for 60 seconds, breathing normally, then proceed to Move 4

a

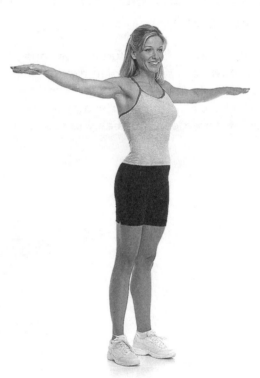

eat nutritionally, *not* emotionally® visualization

Today you are going to use visualization to help build your inner gratitude. Once you build gratitude, you'll more easily be able to handle any negative emotions that may have led to overeating in the past. Close your eyes and take a few deep, relaxing breaths, in through your nose and out through your mouth. Every time you exhale, allow your body to grow more and more relaxed. Once you feel completely relaxed, you are ready to start.

MOVE 4: high heel hold
calves

a. Stand with your feet directly under your hips. Exhale as you lift your heels, rising onto the balls of your feet. Pretend you are wearing very high heels. (Place one hand on a chair or wall for balance, if needed.) Hold for 60 seconds, breathing normally. Release and return to Move 1 on page 98. Repeat Moves 1–4 once more and you're done.

a

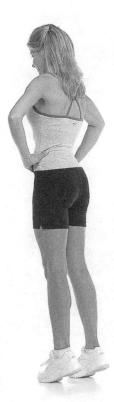

in praise of you

Reflect on your good qualities. First, start with what you do well. Are you a good friend or mother? Reflect on how you affect others in your life. What good things have you done in your life? Remember in every detail the good acts you've done. You might remember the birth of your child or a good deed you did for someone in need. Recall a time when you were instrumental in making someone else happy. Recall every detail of that memory. For the next few moments, continue to dwell on details in your past when you lived up to your expectations for yourself. Realize that you have done more good than bad in this world. Allow yourself to feel grateful for yourself. Allow this gratitude to grow in your heart.

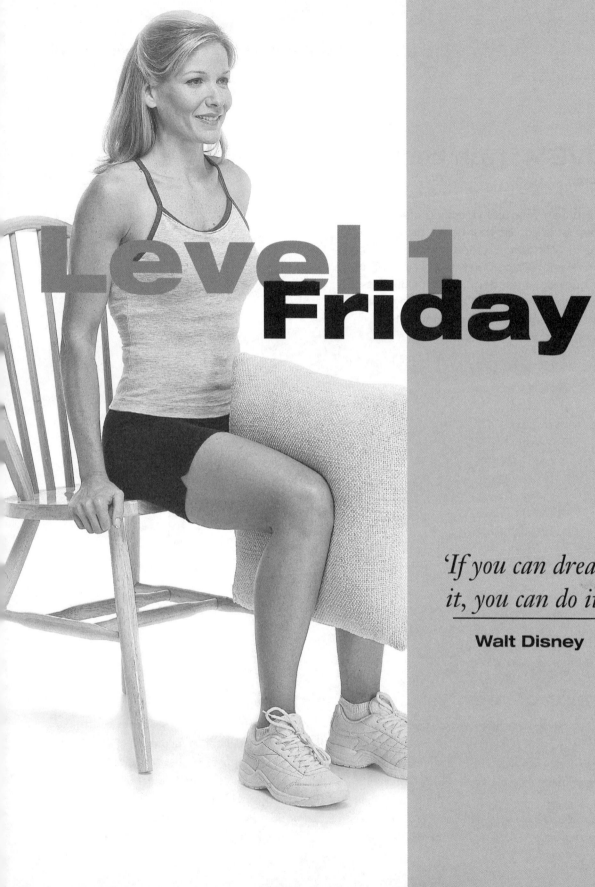

Level 1
Friday

'If you can dream it, you can do it.'

Walt Disney

jorge's power thought

Do you wish you could see what your future body will look like? Do you want to know what you will look like with leaner hips and thinner thighs? Some of my clients relied on photos of their youth – photos taken before they gained weight in their trouble zones – to help motivate them toward their goal. But I've found a better way. You can see your future body *today*, with the help of the World Wide Web.

A wonderful online tool will help you to create a photo of yourself at your future goal. It uses photo technology created by a company in Canada called MyVirtualModel. Go to www.myvirtualmodel.com and simply follow the online directions and soon you'll see the future you – with leaner hips and thinner thighs. Then print out the photos and put them on your refrigerator to motivate you to stick with the programme.

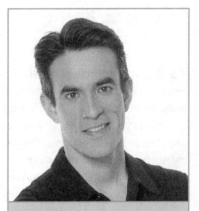

'Your photos of your future body will serve as a powerful motivating force. They will help keep you motivated and focused.'

8 minute moves®
thighs day

MOVE 1: seated pillow squeeze
inner thighs

a. Sit on a sturdy chair (one without wheels). Rest your feet on the floor with your knees bent at 90-degree angles. Place a pillow between your thighs. Exhale as you squeeze the pillow between your thighs, as if you were trying to squeeze the stuffing out of the pillow. Hold for 1 minute as you breathe normally. Release and proceed to Move 2.

a

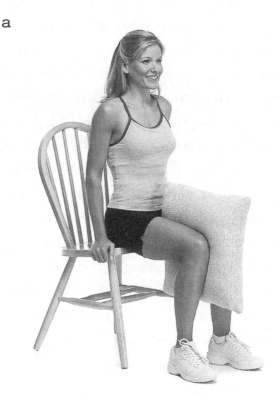

8-MINUTE LOG				
exercise	move 1	move 2	move 3	move 4
sets				
reps				

MOVE 2: seated hand push
outer thighs and hips

a. Sit on a sturdy chair. Rest your feet on the floor with your knees bent at 90-degree angles. Place your palms on the outsides of your knees. While keeping your palms and arms stationary, push your knees outward against your palms, as if you were trying to push your palms away. At the same time, press inward with your hands, preventing your thighs from pushing them outward. Hold this isometric contraction for 1 minute, breathing normally. Release and proceed to Move 3 on page 106.

a

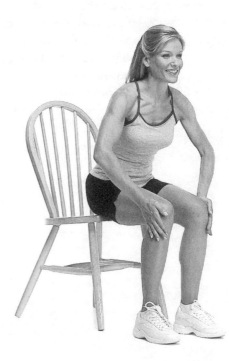

exercise sequence

1. warm up Jog or march on the spot for 1 minute.

2. cruise moves Do one 60-second repetition of each of your 4 Cruise Moves. Repeat this cycle and you will be done in 8 minutes.

3. cool down After your Cruise Moves, do these stretches (see page 74).

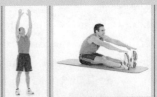

Sky-reaching pose | Hurdler's stretch | Cobra stretch

thighs day (cont'd)

MOVE 3: seated leg raise
fronts of the thighs

a. Sit on a sturdy chair. Rest your feet on the floor with your knees bent at 90-degree angles. Rest your hands on the chair at your sides. Exhale as you lift and extend your right leg. Hold for 30 seconds as you breathe normally. Then inhale as you lower your right leg and exhale as you repeat with your left leg. Hold for 30 seconds while breathing normally. Release and proceed to Move 4.

a

eat nutritionally, *not* emotionally®
visualization

Today you are going to build so much love that your heart overflows, allowing you to share that love with others – even people you don't know that well! Once you fill up your own heart with love, it's so much easier to bring joy and peace to the lives of others. It's also so much easier to deal with difficult people who, in the past, may have caused you to plunge into a bad mood.

Start by taking a few deep, relaxing breaths, in through your nose and out through your mouth. Once you feel deeply relaxed, you're ready to begin.

MOVE 4: seated bridge
backs of the thighs and rear end

a. Sit on the edge of a sturdy chair. Rest your feet on the floor with your knees bent at 90-degree angles. Rest your palms on the chair at your sides. Exhale as you lift your hips, allowing your palms and feet to support your body weight. Continue to lift your hips until your body resembles the shape of a bridge. Hold for 20 to 60 seconds while breathing normally. Release and return to Move 1 on page 104. Repeat Moves 1–4 once more and you're done.

a

overflowing love

Visualize a warm, white, loving energy growing in your heart. Feel this energy expand, filling up every space in your heart and making you feel content.

Visualize a person who needs help. It might be someone you know through work or someone who lives in your neighbourhood or even in your house. Allow yourself to feel any pain or suffering that this person might be feeling. Then, see the loving energy that you've created in your heart expand beyond your body and enter this person. See the energy fill their heart and wash away negativity. See the loving energy completely heal them of worry, mistrust, and anger. Feel good about yourself for helping someone else in need.

Level 1
Saturday

'It is never too late to be what you might have been.'

George Eliot

jorge's power thought

Today is your day off from Cruise Moves. Tomorrow you will also take the day off. Use this time to relax from your Cruise Moves.

Relaxation is just as important as exercise; it helps give your mind an important break. When you relax, you turn on your parasympathetic nervous system. This nervous system is the opposite of the one that governs your actions during the week. All too often we spend most of our time during the work week in a state of agitation, with our fight-or-flight response turned on. You must turn off your fight-or-flight response and turn on your parasympathetic nervous system from time to time. If you don't, your body and mind will become burned out. You'll feel irritable and fatigued. When you feel tired, you won't want to tackle your Cruise Moves.

I know some of you will feel guilty when you relax. You will think, 'I know I should be doing something'. When such guilty thoughts pop into your head, just use the 'Oops' technique you learned earlier. Say 'Oops' out loud and return to lounging in the garden.

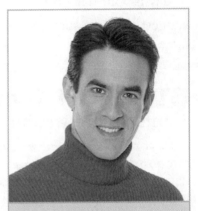

'Every good thing you do for your body – even relaxing – will help you reach your goal more quickly.'

stretches
day off from cruise moves

Today is your day off from your Cruise Moves. To accelerate your results, I suggest that you spend 8 minutes this morning stretching and lengthening your muscles.

STRETCH 1: thigh lengthener
fronts of the thighs

a. Lie on your left side with your legs extended. Support your upper torso on your left forearm. Bend your right leg, grasping your foot with your right hand. Exhale as you use your hand to gently pull your right foot toward your buttocks as you simultaneously tuck in your tailbone and flatten the natural arch in your lower spine. Once in position, breathe normally as you hold the stretch for 30 seconds. Release and repeat on the other side. Then proceed to Stretch 2.

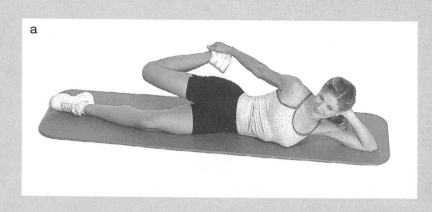

eat nutritionally, *not* emotionally®
visualization

During your last visualization, you shared your love with someone else. During this visualization, you will learn how to cultivate love toward those whom you experience difficulty getting along with. Close your eyes and take a few deep, relaxing breaths, in through your nose and out through your mouth. Allow each exhalation to bring you to a state of deep relaxation. Once you feel deeply relaxed, you're ready to begin.

STRETCH 2: seated forward bend
outer thighs and hips

a. Sit on the floor. Cross your legs so that your right foot rests in the crease made by your bent left knee and your right leg rests on top of your left leg, forming a triangle with your legs.

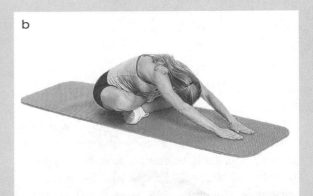

b. Inhale as you lengthen your spine. Exhale as you bend forward from the hips. Once in position, breathe normally, holding the stretch for 30 seconds. Then inhale as you rise to the starting position. Rearrange your legs so that your left leg is on top and repeat. Then proceed to Stretch 3 on page 112.

loving your enemies

See in your mind the image of a person with whom you experience difficulty getting along. Rather than focusing on this person's negative qualities, however, I want you to focus on what makes this person endearing. At first, this may be difficult, but visualize this person's good qualities and virtues. Perhaps this person is understanding or a good listener or a hard worker. Try to remember a time when you got along with this person. Perhaps she was kind to you during a time of stress. Cultivate this memory in your mind and try to call up every detail. As you do so, feel a sense of love growing in your heart. End your visualization by wishing that this person stay free from suffering. You'll be surprised by how much your positive wishes affect your relationship for the better!

stretches
day off from cruise moves (cont'd)

STRETCH 3: hamstring stretch
backs of the thighs

a. Lie on your back with your knees bent and feet on the floor. Lift your left leg, bringing your knee in toward your chest. Wrap a towel around the arch of your left foot, holding the ends of the towel in your hands.

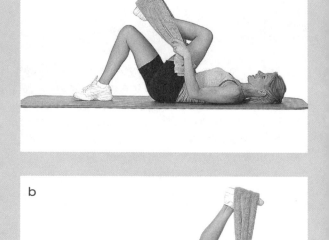

b. Exhale as you extend your leg toward the ceiling. Use your hands to gently pull your foot toward your face. Breathe normally as you hold for 30 seconds. Lower your leg and repeat on the other side. Then proceed to Stretch 4.

STRETCH 4: frog
inner thighs

a. Start in a table position with your knees under your hips and hands under your shoulders. Widen your knees 15–30 cm (6–12 in) and turn your toes outward.

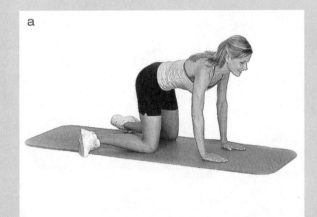

b. Exhale as you gently bring your hips back toward your feet, feeling a stretch in your inner thighs and groin. Once in position, hold for 60 seconds as you breathe normally. Then release and return to Stretch 1 on page 110. Repeat Stretches 1–4 once more, and you're done.

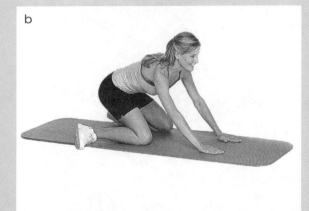

Level 1
Sunday

'Nothing great
was ever
achieved without
enthusiasm.'

**Ralph Waldo
Emerson**

jorge's power thought

Today is your day off from your Cruise Moves. I encourage you to spend the extra 8 minutes today preparing for the week to come. Flip through cookbooks or your recipe collection and pick some meals for the week. Then create your shopping list.

Write down the meals you plan to eat during the week, particularly lunch and dinner. Pencil these meals into your day planner, along with the time that you plan to eat them. If you need to do anything to make sure that meal happens – like popping out to the supermarket in your lunch hour – pencil in that task as well.

You also might spend more time in the kitchen by chopping up some veggies to eat during the week. Or you might cook up some food during the day and create your own homemade frozen dinners. Use Sunday as your planning day. It will help you to stay on track.

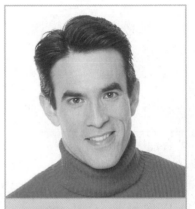

'Follow the Boy Scout motto and be prepared. A little extra preparation on Sundays can make the rest of your week flow so much more easily.'

capture your progress
day off from cruise moves

Today is your day off. Take a moment to relish your progress. Grab a pen and answer the following questions.

1. What is your current weight?

_____

2. What was your original weight?

_____

3. What is your waist circumference?

_____

4. What was your original waist circumference?

_____

5. What have you done well this week? What are you most proud of?

_____

_____

_____

_____

_____

_____

6. What could you improve next week?

_____

_____

_____

_____

_____

_____

eat nutritionally, *not* emotionally® visualization

One of the first steps to eliminating emotional eating begins with you. It begins with treating yourself with the utmost respect, and you can do that only if you love yourself and your body. Sometimes cultivating self-love in the place of self-hate can be difficult. Today, you will complete a visualization that will help. Close your eyes and take a few deep, relaxing breaths, in through your nose and out through your mouth. Allow each exhalation to bring you to a state of deep relaxation. Once you feel completely relaxed, you're ready to begin.

cheryl lost 9 cm (3½ in) off her thighs!

'The best part of the Jorge Cruise® programme is the minimal amount of time involved. It fits perfectly into my morning routine. I am able to get up from bed, get on the floor, and, before I realize that I am actually exercising, it's over! And I still get the benefits. For the amount of time involved – 8 minutes – you have to be just plain lazy not to try it.

My results have inspired me to move even more. I am more active overall and I feel that I want to be outdoors doing things like walking and riding my bike. I have more energy and don't find myself sitting around as much. I've truly changed my lifestyle for the better.'

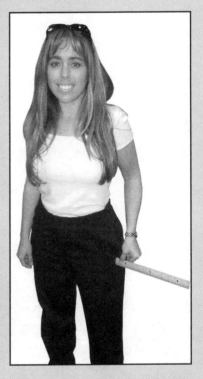

Cheryl slimmed down her thighs and lost nearly 6 kg (13 lb).

cultivating inner love

Think back to a time in your life when you felt good about yourself. Perhaps you accomplished something significant, won an award, or got a promotion at work. Whatever it was, bring the memory of that happy time fully into your awareness.

See every detail of that moment. Try to feel the emotions you felt. Think back to the smells, sights, sounds and sensations of that moment. Try to recall it as vividly as possible.

Take a few moments to relish the good feeling that you've just created inside of yourself. Know that these positive feelings are always there inside of you, waiting to be called upon at any moment.

Level 2
Monday

'There came a time
when the risk to
remain tight in a
bud was more
painful than the
risk it took to
blossom.'

Anaïs Nin

jorge's power thought

Many people ask me why I suggest you perform each Cruise Move for 60 seconds. Besides the fact that it allows your Cruise Move session to total a nice and neat 8 minutes, I do have some other, more important reasons. I didn't pick 60 seconds out of thin air!

Some resistance-training programmes require you to count repetitions, suggesting that you lift a weight 12 to 15 times. My first book did this. I've found in working with millions of clients that simply watching the clock is sometimes an easier way to move! It frees your mind from counting and forces you to fully fatigue the muscle you are working. It's super simple and convenient.

But why 60 seconds? I've found with much trial and error that 60 seconds is the ideal amount of time needed to start firming your muscles. In testing my Jorge Cruise® programmes on client after client, they loved it and saw the results!

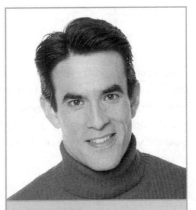

'I learned my most important lessons about weight loss from people just like you.'

8 minute moves®
thighs day

MOVE 1: standing leg swing
inner thighs

a. Stand next to a chair or wall, placing your left hand on the chair or wall for support. Your feet should be directly under your hips. Shift your body weight over your left foot. Inhale as you lift your right foot off the floor and outward slightly.

b. Exhale as you swing your right foot to the left, in front of and past your left leg. Hold for a count of 2. Inhale as you return to the starting position. Repeat for 30 seconds. Switch legs and repeat for 30 seconds, then proceed to Move 2.

a

b

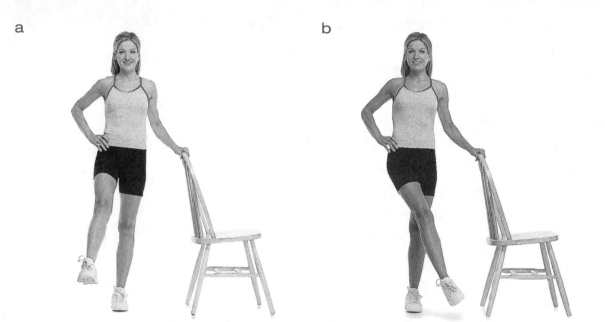

8-MINUTE LOG				
exercise	move 1	move 2	move 3	move 4
sets				
reps				

MOVE 2: standing side raise
outer thighs and hips

a. Stand next to a chair or wall, placing your left hand on the chair or wall for support. Your feet should be directly under your hips. Shift your body weight over your left foot. Exhale as you lift and extend your right leg laterally away from your torso as far as you can. Hold for a count of 2. Inhale as you return to the starting position. Repeat for 30 seconds. Switch legs and repeat for 30 seconds, then proceed to Move 3 on page 122.

a

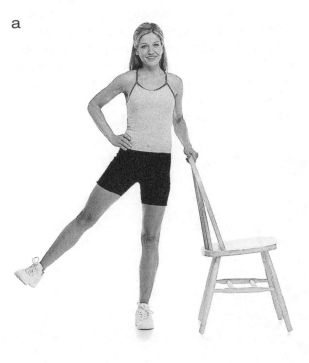

exercise sequence

1. warm up Jog or march on the spot for 1 minute.

2. cruise moves Do one 60-second repetition of each of your 4 Cruise Moves. Repeat this cycle and you will be done in 8 minutes.

3. cool down After your Cruise Moves, do these stretches (see page 74).

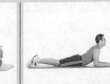

Sky-reaching pose | **Hurdler's stretch** | **Cobra stretch**

thighs day (cont'd)

MOVE 3: standing knee lift
fronts of the thighs

a. Stand next to a chair or wall, placing your right hand on the chair or wall for support. Your feet should be directly under your hips. Shift your body weight over your right foot. Exhale as you lift your left knee, until your left thigh is parallel with the floor. Hold for a count of 2. Inhale and release. Repeat for 30 seconds. Switch legs, repeat for 30 seconds, and then proceed to Move 4.

a

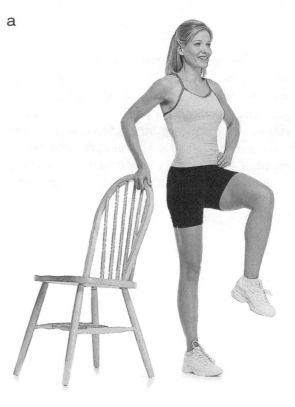

eat nutritionally, *not* emotionally®
visualization

For today's visualization, I'd like you to explore your own passion and see where it will take you. You'll find that you can use your passion as a powerful motivating force. It will help you stick with your new health habits. Close your eyes and take a few deep, relaxing breaths, in through your nose and out through your mouth. Allow each exhalation to bring you to a state of deep relaxation. Once you feel completely relaxed, you're ready to begin.

MOVE 4: standing leg lift
backs of the thighs and rear end

a. Stand facing a chair or wall. Place one or both hands against the chair or wall for support. Shift your body weight over your left foot. Exhale as you lift and extend your right leg behind your torso as high as you can. Be careful not to overarch your lower back as you do so. Hold for a count of 2. Inhale and release. Repeat for 30 seconds. Switch legs, repeat, and then return to Move 1 on page 120. Repeat Moves 1–4 once more and you're done.

a

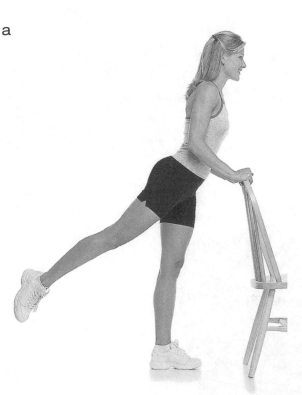

unleash your inner passion

Visualize yourself 1 year in the future. See yourself as you would like to be. You are accomplishing all of the things that you wanted in life with strength and vigour. You are focusing on what's most important to you and making your mark on the world.

What new mental, physical and spiritual qualities have you uncovered? What lessons have you learned? What did you develop inside of yourself to be able to accomplish so much? What was most important in helping you to achieve success? What helped you overcome any challenges along the way?

With those answers, return to the present moment and visualize what you must do right now to make your future become reality.

Level 2
Tuesday

'The great dividing
line between success
and failure can be
expressed in five
words, "I did not
have time."'

Franklin Field

jorge's power thought

As you progress along your journey to lean hips and thin thighs, it may help to revisit the reason you started this journey in the first place. Have you ever known someone who was so passionate and so focused that nothing could stand in his or her way? Usually such passion comes from having a very clear plan – a mental blueprint – that guides you successfully towards your goal.

To ignite your passion for leaner hips and thinner thighs, take a moment to think about what you want your new, dream body to look like. You might even take out a piece of paper and jot down some notes. Write down not only how you want your hips and thighs to look, but also how you want them to feel. Also write down what you'd like others to notice about your hips and thighs. And even write down what types of clothes you might wear or feel more comfortable wearing once you reach your dream goal.

Whenever you feel like you need an extra bit of motivation, you can turn to the list you just created to remind yourself *why* you decided to take this journey. Remember: it's well worth the effort.

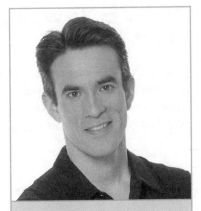

'With a clear target, you have the most powerful advantage to making your dream body a reality.'

8 minute moves®
upper-body day

MOVE 1: wall pump
chest

a. Stand arm's length away from a wall with your feet directly under your hips. Lean forward and place your palms against the wall. Your elbows should be slightly bent.

b. Inhale as you slowly bend your elbows, bringing your chest and torso closer to the wall. Exhale as you slowly press yourself back to the starting position, straightening your arms as you go. Slowly repeat for 60 seconds. Release and proceed to Move 2.

a

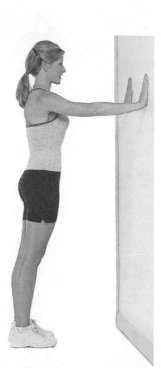

b

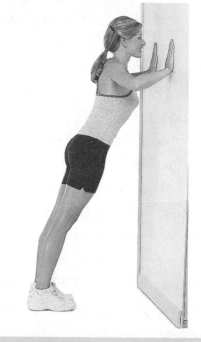

8-MINUTE LOG				
exercise	move 1	move 2	move 3	move 4
sets				
reps				

MOVE 2: posture pump
upper back

a. Stand with your heels, buttocks and head against a wall or sturdy, closed door. Rest your arms comfortably at your sides.

b. Exhale as you pull your upper back and shoulders toward the wall, flattening everything from your ribs to your shoulders against the wall. Get your lower back as close as possible to the wall as you can. Relax and repeat for 60 seconds. Proceed to Move 3 on page 128.

a

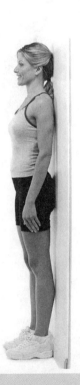

b

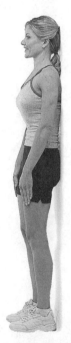

exercise sequence

1. warm up Jog or march on the spot for 1 minute.

2. cruise moves Do one 60-second repetition of each of your 4 Cruise Moves. Repeat this cycle and you will be done in 8 minutes.

3. cool down After your Cruise Moves, do these stretches (see page 74).

Sky-reaching pose | Hurdler's stretch | Cobra stretch

upper-body day (cont'd)

MOVE 3: book hold
biceps

a. Stand with your feet directly under your hips. Balance a heavy textbook or phone book in each hand with your palms facing up and your arms bent at 90 degrees. Hold for 60 seconds as you breathe normally, keeping your back long and straight and your abdominals firm. Release and proceed to Move 4.

a

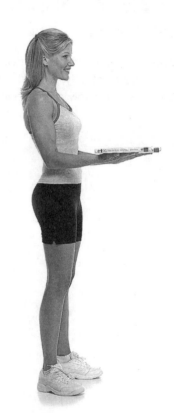

eat nutritionally, *not* emotionally®
visualization

Visualization can help you to face life's little challenges with more ease. Instead of problems, you see solutions. Instead of turning to food, you can turn to your mind for help. When life throws you a lemon, you can easily turn it into lemonade! Let's use visualization to help you turn your first lemon into *lemonaid*, shall we? Close your eyes and take a few deep, relaxing breaths, in through your nose and out through your mouth. Allow each exhalation to bring you to a state of deep relaxation. Once you feel completely relaxed, you're ready to begin.

MOVE 4: kickback hold
triceps

a. Stand with your feet directly under your hips. Bend forward from your hips about 45 degrees with your arms extended.

b. Exhale as you lift your extended arms up behind your torso. Stop once you've lifted your arms as high as possible without locking your elbows. Hold for 60 seconds, breathing normally. Release and return to Move 1 on page 126. Repeat Moves 1–4 once more and you're done.

a

b

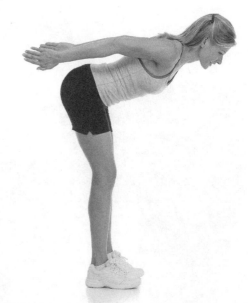

mental lemonade

You're driving home when suddenly, you hear a 'clunk, clunk, clunk' sound as your car begins to bounce around. It's a flat tyre! Instead of panicking, you calmly steer your car to the side of the road and turn on your hazard lights. Carefully you open your door and get out to assess the situation and then go to your boot and retrieve the spare tyre, car jack and wheel brace. See yourself loosening the wheel nuts, and positioning the jack. You use strong, solid, even strokes on the jack and up your car goes! You remove the flat tyre and hoist it back in your trunk, install the spare, replace the wheel nuts, lower your car and go on your way. How do you feel knowing that you can overcome any obstacle that comes your way?

Level 2
Wednesday

'The best time
to plant a tree was
20 years ago.
The second best
time is now.'

Chinese proverb

jorge's power thought

All of us have what I like to call a loser zone, a place where we spend too much of our time. You fall into a loser zone when you do something that produces no significant improvement in your life. The number one loser zone activity? Watching television. When you watch TV, you're not only sedentary – and therefore burning very few calories – but you are also more likely to eat mindlessly. Commercials that depict food will make you crave food when you are not truly hungry.

Other loser zones include aimlessly chatting on the phone and surfing the Internet. What are your loser zones and how many hours a day do you spend losing precious time? I'm not suggesting that you should be on the go all the time. As I've said before, relaxation is very important. However, if you spend more than 6 to 8 hours a week in loser zone activities, you have just found some time that could be better spent focusing on your hips and thighs!

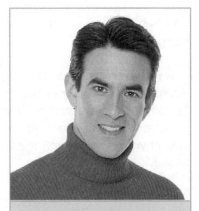

'Shrink your loser zones and you'll maximize the time you have to spend fighting your trouble zones.'

8 minute moves®
thighs day

MOVE 1: standing leg swing
inner thighs

a. Stand next to a chair or wall, placing your left hand on the chair or wall for support. Your feet should be directly under your hips. Shift your body weight over your left foot. Inhale as you lift your right foot off the floor and outward slightly.

b. Exhale as you swing your right foot to the left, in front of and past your left leg. Hold for a count of 2. Inhale as you return to the starting position. Repeat for 30 seconds. Switch legs and repeat for 30 seconds, then proceed to Move 2.

a

b

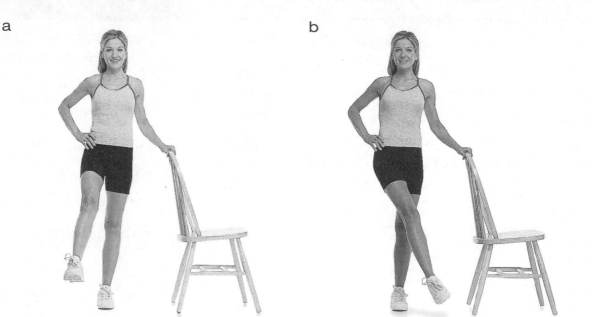

8-MINUTE LOG				
exercise	move 1	move 2	move 3	move 4
sets				
reps				

MOVE 2: standing side raise
outer thighs and hips

a. Stand next to a chair or wall, placing your left hand on the chair or wall for support. Your feet should be directly under your hips. Shift your body weight over your left foot. Exhale as you lift and extend your right leg laterally away from your torso as far as you can. Hold for a count of 2. Inhale as you return to the starting position. Repeat for 30 seconds. Switch legs and repeat for 30 seconds, then proceed to Move 3 on page 134.

a

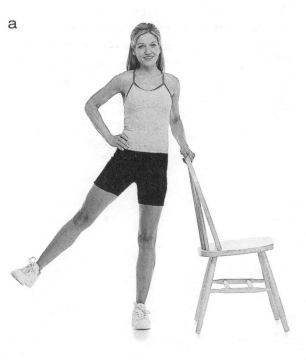

exercise sequence

1. warm up Jog or march on the spot for 1 minute.

2. cruise moves Do one 60-second repetition of each of your 4 Cruise Moves. Repeat this cycle and you will be done in 8 minutes.

3. cool down After your Cruise Moves, do these stretches (see page 74).

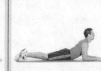

Sky-reaching pose | **Hurdler's stretch** | **Cobra stretch**

thighs day (cont'd)

MOVE 3: standing knee lift
fronts of the thighs

a. Stand next to a chair or wall, placing your right hand on the chair or wall for support. Your feet should be directly under your hips. Shift your body weight over your right foot. Exhale as you lift your left knee, until your left thigh is parallel with the floor. Hold for a count of 2. Inhale and release. Repeat for 30 seconds. Switch legs, repeat for 30 seconds, and then proceed to Move 4.

a

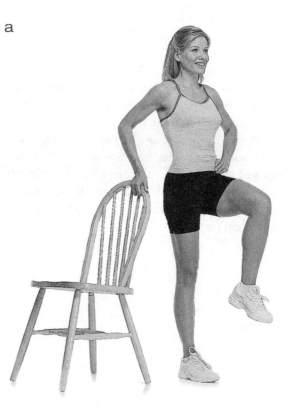

eat nutritionally, *not* emotionally®
visualization

For today's visualization, you will again use the power of your mind to help you solve problems that might have led to emotional eating in the past. Today you will use visualization to help you overcome the urge to eat when you encounter difficult people. Take a few moments to relax by taking a few deep breaths, in through your nose and out through your mouth. Feel each exhalation relax you more and more deeply. Once you are fully relaxed, you are ready to begin.

MOVE 4: standing leg lift
backs of the thighs and rear end

a. Stand facing a chair or wall. Place one or both hands against the chair or wall for support. Shift your body weight over your left foot. Exhale as you lift and extend your right leg behind your torso as high as you can. Be careful not to overarch your lower back as you do so. Hold for a count of 2. Inhale and release. Repeat for 30 seconds. Switch legs, repeat, and then return to Move 1 on page 132. Repeat Moves 1–4 once more and you're done.

a
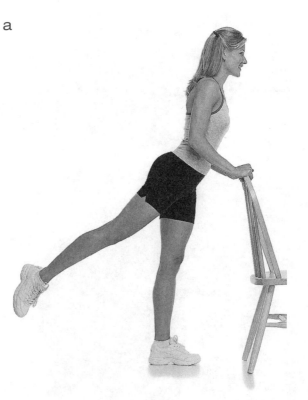

seeing your problems vanish

Imagine someone with whom you may be having some personal conflict. It might be your spouse or your child or someone at work. Bring the image of that person into your mind. Imagine having a positive interaction with that person. Start with some small talk. See yourself confronting this person about what is bothering you. See yourself calmly, nicely and succinctly voicing your concerns, keeping the focus on how this person makes you feel. See this person respond positively. You will soon find that if you mentally see yourself confronting your problems, you won't feel so much stress or anxiety when you try to solve them in real life!

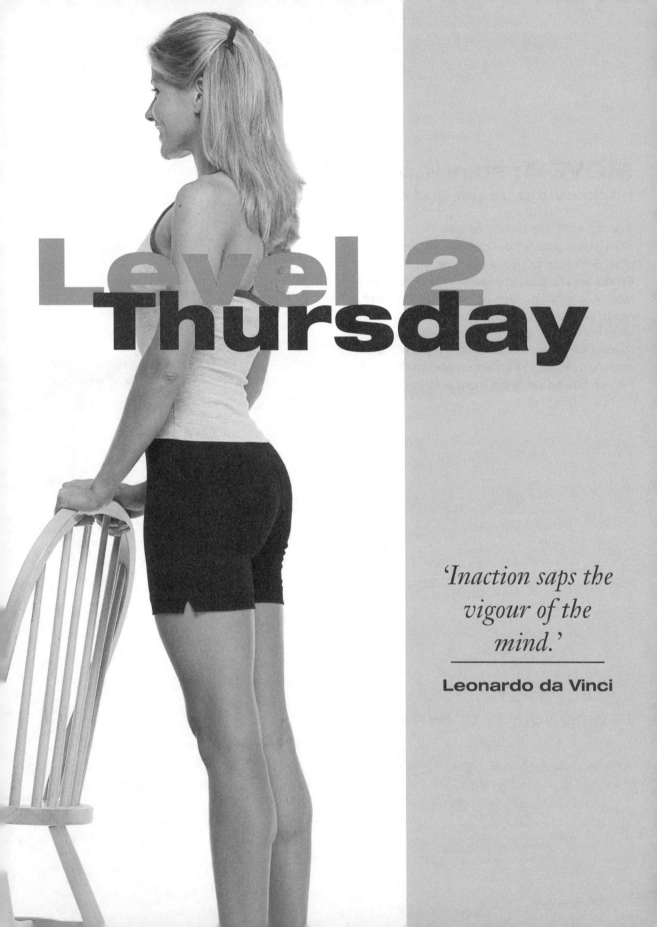

Level 2
Thursday

'Inaction saps the
vigour of the
mind.'

Leonardo da Vinci

jorge's power thought

Many people ask me for secrets on getting out of bed in the morning. They tell me that they are not a morning person, and that they just can't exercise as soon as they jump out of bed.

I always share this simple trick. To help jump start your morning, do the following as soon as the alarm goes off. Sit up in bed and bring your hands together for a strong clap. With every breath, clap strongly. The palms of your hands have more nerve receptors than almost any other part of your body. Clapping your hands creates a neurological jolt that literally stimulates your brain. Then jump out of bed and stand up with good posture. Bring your shoulders back and your chest out. This will activate your diaphragm muscle (located under your lungs), which helps maximize your oxygen intake. Then jog on the spot. That will get your heart pumping.

Trust me on this one. If you do that simple technique, you'll be out of bed and ready for your Cruise Moves in no time.

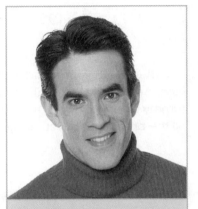

'An extra hour of sleep will help to reset your body clock, allowing you to wake up refreshed.'

8 minute moves®
torso and calves day

MOVE 1: belly breath pump
belly

a. Stand with your feet directly under your hips. As you exhale, contract and press your tummy muscles inward as you slowly squeeze all the breath out of your lungs.

b. Reverse the motion by relaxing your tummy outward to slowly pull air into your lungs. Repeat for 1 minute, fully emptying and filling your lungs. Then proceed to Move 2.

a

b

8-MINUTE LOG				
exercise	move 1	move 2	move 3	move 4
sets				
reps				

MOVE 2: superman
lower back

a. Lie with your belly on the floor, your legs straight and your arms extended in front of you, like Superman flying through the air. Exhale as you simultaneously lift your arms and legs about 10 cm (4 in) off the floor. If you begin to feel pinching in your lower back, focus on lengthening your spine by reaching out through your fingertips and toes. Also, make sure your head remains in a neutral position with your gaze at the floor. Hold for 1 minute and then proceed to Move 3 on page 140.

a

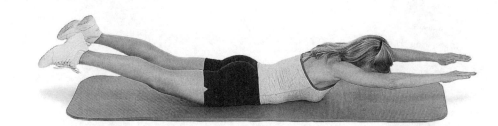

exercise sequence

1. warm up Jog or march on the spot for 1 minute.

2. cruise moves Do one 60-second repetition of each of your 4 Cruise Moves. Repeat this cycle and you will be done in 8 minutes.

3. cool down After your Cruise Moves, do these stretches (see page 74).

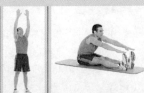

Sky-reaching pose | **Hurdler's stretch** | **Cobra stretch**

torso and calves day (cont'd)

MOVE 3: bird pump
shoulders

a. Stand with your feet directly under your hips and your arms resting at your sides. Raise and extend your arms about 45 degrees out from your hips. Make sure your shoulders are relaxed, your tummy is firm and your upper back straight.

b. Exhale as you raise your arms about 45 degrees above shoulder level. Inhale as you lower them to the starting position. Slowly repeat for 1 minute. Release and proceed to Move 4.

a

b

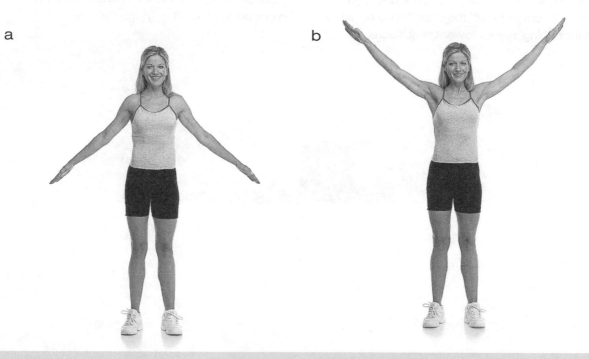

eat nutritionally, *not* emotionally®
visualization

Many of my clients tell me that they are most likely to overeat when they feel worthless or 'not good enough'. Today's visualization will help you to overcome such feelings. Today you will cultivate your inner self-love. Close your eyes and take a few deep, relaxing breaths, in through your nose and out through your mouth. Once you feel completely relaxed, you are ready to begin.

MOVE 4: standing calf pump
calves

a. Stand next to a sturdy chair or wall with your feet directly under your hips and your arms resting at your sides. Place one hand on the chair or wall for balance.

b. Exhale as you rise onto the balls of your feet, bringing your heels off the floor. Inhale as you lower your heels back to the floor. Repeat for 1 minute, then return to Move 1 on page 138. Repeat Moves 1–4 once more and you're done.

a

b

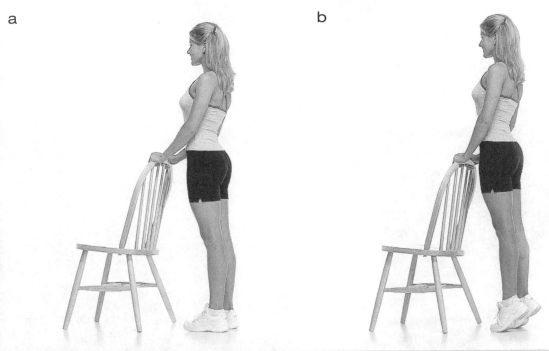

you at centre stage

See yourself through the eyes of someone else, someone who really cares about you, such as a close friend, a spouse, or one of your children. Feel the same admiration that this person feels as you watch yourself through their eyes. Try to see all of the good qualities about yourself that *they* see every day. Watch yourself as your loved ones walk up to you and tell you how much they love and admire you. Watch your expression as they tell you about your good qualities. What do they say? Now imagine more and more people coming into the room and staring at you with the same love and admiration as your loved one. As the room fills with people, they begin to applaud, clapping for you!

Level 2
Friday

'You should plant your own garden instead of waiting for someone else to bring you flowers.'

Veronica Shoffstall

jorge's power thought

Many people ask me whether they can skip their cooldown. They tell me that stretching won't help them create leaner hips and thinner thighs, so why bother? Well, that's simply not true.

Stretching helps you accomplish your goal in a number of ways. Most important, stretching helps increase *flexibility*, which, in turn, helps your muscles to grow stronger. Yes, it's true! Researchers have found that flexible muscles tend to be stronger and more aerobic than tight muscles. Also, stretching will help to **lengthen your muscles,** creating a long, lean appearance. Finally, it helps to bring circulation to your muscles, allowing them to more quickly recover from your Cruise Moves. This circulation is also important in preventing cellulite. So keep stretching!

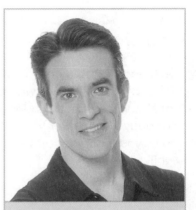

'Your cooldown will help prepare your body to face the day, allowing you to feel refreshed.'

8 minute moves®
thighs day

MOVE 1: standing leg swing
inner thighs

a. Stand next to a chair or wall, placing your left hand on the chair or wall for support. Your feet should be directly under your hips. Shift your body weight over your left foot. Inhale as you lift your right foot off the floor and outward slightly.

b. Exhale as you swing your right foot to the left, in front of and past your left leg. Hold for a count of 2. Inhale as you return to the starting position. Repeat for 30 seconds. Switch legs and repeat for 30 seconds, then proceed to Move 2.

a

b

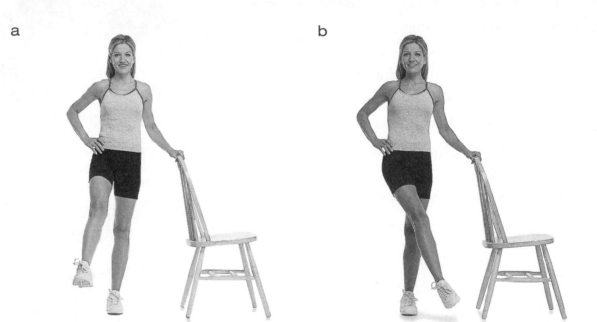

8-MINUTE LOG				
exercise	move 1	move 2	move 3	move 4
sets				
reps				

MOVE 2: standing side raise
outer thighs and hips

a. Stand next to a chair or wall, placing your left hand on the chair or wall for support. Your feet should be directly under your hips. Shift your body weight over your left foot. Exhale as you lift and extend your right leg laterally away from your torso as far as you can. Hold for a count of 2. Inhale as you return to the starting position. Repeat for 30 seconds. Switch legs and repeat for 30 seconds, then proceed to Move 3 on page 146.

a

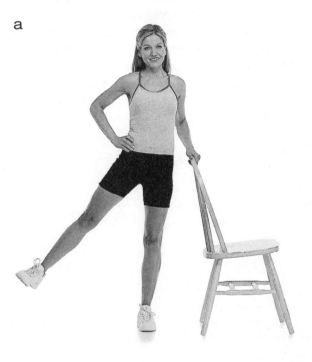

exercise sequence

1. warm up Jog or march on the spot for 1 minute.

2. cruise moves Do one 60-second repetition of each of your 4 Cruise Moves. Repeat this cycle and you will be done in 8 minutes.

3. cool down After your Cruise Moves, do these stretches (see page 74).

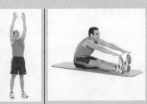

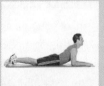

Sky-reaching pose | Hurdler's stretch | Cobra stretch

thighs day (cont'd)

MOVE 3: standing knee lift
fronts of the thighs

a. Stand next to a chair or wall, placing your right hand on the chair or wall for support. Your feet should be directly under your hips. Shift your body weight over your right foot. Exhale as you lift your left knee, until your left thigh is parallel with the floor. Hold for a count of 2. Inhale and release. Repeat for 30 seconds. Switch legs, repeat for 30 seconds, and then proceed to Move 4.

a

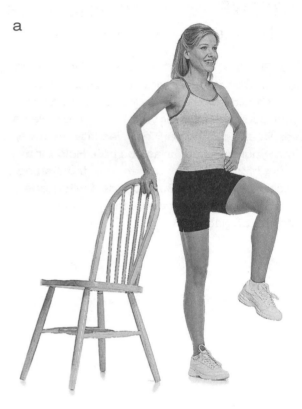

eat nutritionally, *not* emotionally® visualization

Today you will again use the power of visualization to help you to better deal the emotions that may arise from encounters with difficult people. Close your eyes and take a few deep, relaxing breaths, in through your nose and out through your mouth. Allow each exhalation to relax you more deeply. Once you feel completely relaxed, you are ready to begin.

MOVE 4: standing leg lift
backs of the thighs and rear end

a. Stand facing a chair or wall. Place one or both hands against the chair or wall for support. Shift your body weight over your left foot. Exhale as you lift and extend your right leg behind your torso as high as you can. Be careful not to overarch your lower back as you do so. Hold for a count of 2. Inhale and release. Repeat for 30 seconds. Switch legs, repeat, and then return to Move 1 on page 144. Repeat Moves 1–4 once more and you're done.

a

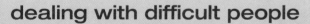

dealing with difficult people

Think of someone who usually makes you feel a negative emotion. If the image of this person makes you feel very angry, sad, or anxious, take a few deep, relaxing breaths to help yourself return to a more relaxed state. Then, put yourself in this person's shoes. Try to imagine what a typical day in this person's life must be like. Experience every encounter and every emotion. Imagine how you would feel if you lived the same life as this person. Imagine how you would like others to respond to you.

After you have finished, notice whether you have any new insights into this person. Notice whether the image of this person evokes the same strong emotions as it did before the visualization.

Level 2
Saturday

'Some people wait
so long for their
ship to come in,
their _pier_ collapses.'

John Goddard

jorge's power thought

I've already told you that you must get enough sleep to allow your muscles to repair themselves. Did you know that a solid night's sleep can also sharpen your mind and lift your spirits? That's right, simply getting enough Zzz's helps make concentration easier, and even improves your ability to learn. This is because the more sleep you get, the more minutes your brain spends in the rapid eye movement (REM) phase of sleep. And REM sleep is crucial for cementing new information into long- and short-term memory. Research suggests that it is during REM sleep that we file away everything we learn.

Getting enough sleep is as important to your overall health as regular exercise and a healthy diet. Sometimes my clients tell me that they have trouble falling asleep at night. They say worrisome thoughts keep them awake. I tell them to try this little trick. Lie on your back and breathe deeply 10 times. Then lie on your right side and breathe deeply 15 times. Then lie on your left side and breathe deeply 20 times…if you don't fall asleep before then, that is!

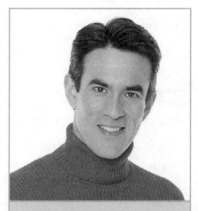

'Try taking a warm bath before bed to soothe away stressful thoughts or tension that might be keeping you awake.'

stretches
day off from cruise moves

Today is your day off from your Cruise Moves. To accelerate your results, I suggest that you spend 8 minutes this morning stretching and lengthening your muscles.

STRETCH 1: butt kick
fronts of the thighs

a. Lie on your belly with your legs extended. Bend your left arm and rest your head in the crook created by your arm. Bend your right leg, bringing your right foot toward your buttocks. Reach back with your right hand and grasp your right foot. Exhale as you use your right hand to gently pull your right foot toward your buttocks. Inhale and, to deepen the stretch, exhale as you press your pubic bone downward into the floor, flattening the natural arch in your lower spine. Hold for a few breaths and then release the pelvic tilt and repeat, holding and releasing over and over for 30 seconds. Release and repeat with the other leg, then proceed to Stretch 2.

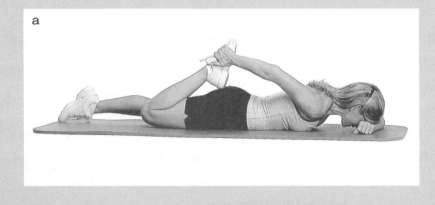

a

eat nutritionally, *not* emotionally®
visualization

Today you will use the power of visualization to help overcome negative feelings that can lead to overeating. You can use this visualization any time you feel a negative mood coming on. Use it whenever you find a negative emotion causing you to think of food.

Start by relaxing with a few deep breaths, in through your nose and out through your mouth. Once you feel deeply relaxed, you are ready to begin.

STRETCH 2: standing hip opener
outer thighs and hips

a. Stand facing a sturdy table. Lift your left thigh in toward your chest, placing your left foot on the tabletop. Turn out your left knee so that your left shin forms a parallel line with the edge of the table. Place your palms on the table for balance.

b. To increase the stretch, lean forward from your hips. Hold for 30 seconds, breathing normally. Switch legs and repeat, then proceed to Stretch 3 on page 152.

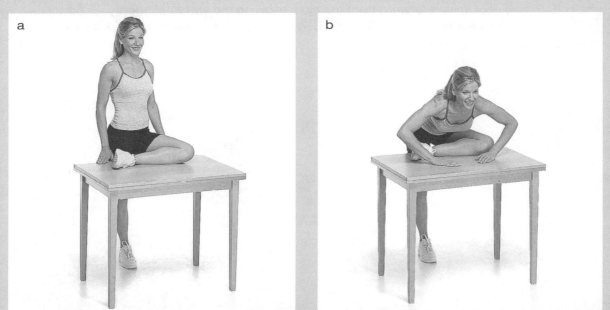

replacing bad with good

Notice the state of your mind. Are you feeling any negative emotions? Do you feel angry, sad, depressed, anxious, or fearful? Each time you exhale, see yourself releasing these negative feelings out of your body. See your breath literally blow them away! Then, each time you inhale, visualize yourself breathing in positive emotions such as love, compassion, joy and peace. With each breath, exchange a negative emotion for a positive one, and feel your body begin to vibrate with positive emotions!

stretches
day off from cruise moves (cont'd)

STRETCH 3: forward bend
backs of the thighs

   a. Stand with your back and buttocks against a wall and your feet about 30 cm (1 ft) in front of the wall. Exhale as you lean forward from the hips, allowing the wall to support your buttocks. Interlace your forearms and relax your upper body. Hold for 60 seconds as you breathe normally. Release and proceed to Stretch 4.

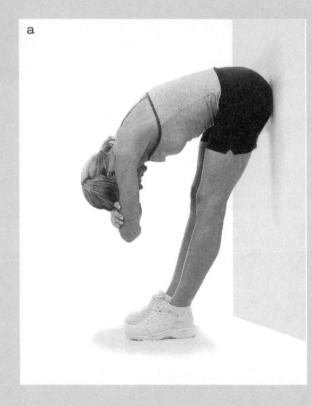

a

STRETCH 4: wide-angle forward bend
inner thighs

a. Stand with your feet about 60–90 cm (2–3 ft) apart. Inhale as you reach your arms overhead. Exhale as you bend forward from your hips, reaching through your fingertips as you bend forward. Try to keep your abs firm and back flat as you bend. Interlace your forearms and relax your upper body. Hold for 60 seconds as you breathe normally. Release and return to Stretch 1 on page 150. Repeat Stretches 1–4 once more, and you're done.

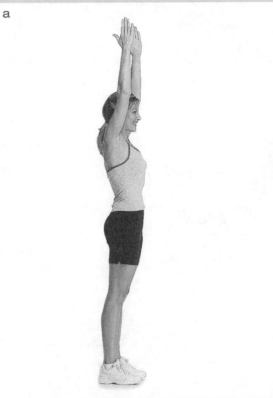

a

Level 2
Sunday

'The greatest discovery of my time is that human beings can alter their lives by altering their attitudes.'

William James

jorge's power thought

Following the Cruise Down Plate will do more than help you avoid overeating. It will also help you eat more fruits and vegetables, many of which are loaded with vitamin C, which plays a very important role in muscle recovery after your Cruise Moves.

This important vitamin helps produce collagen, which is a connective tissue that holds muscles, bones and other tissues together. During exercise, as the rate of your breathing increases to meet the demands of your workout, the chemical interaction of oxygen with your cell membranes, protein, and other cellular components creates damaging substances called free radicals. These free radicals are highly reactive substances that, much like small fires, must be extinguished before they burn, or 'oxidize' neighbouring molecules in other cells, creating muscle soreness and stiffness.

Vitamin C is a dietary antioxidant that helps to put out free radical damage in and around your cells. So follow up your Cruise Moves with a breakfast rich in vitamin C foods such as oranges, red peppers, or cantaloupe.

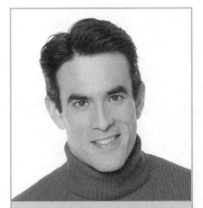

'Brightly coloured fruits and vegetables such as red peppers are packed with vitamin C.'

capture your progress
day off from cruise moves

Today is your day off. Take a moment to relish your progress. Grab a pen and answer the following questions.

1. What is your current weight?
_____

2. What was your original weight?
_____

3. What is your waist circumference?
_____

4. What was your original waist circumference?
_____

5. What have you done well this week? What are you most proud of?
_____
_____
_____
_____
_____
_____

6. What could you improve next week?
_____
_____
_____
_____
_____
_____

eat nutritionally, *not* emotionally®
visualization

Today you will use the power of visualization to help fill yourself up with positive emotions. This visualization is similar to the one you learned on Saturday. You may find that one works better for you than the other. Use whichever one works best for you to help transform bad moods into good ones.

Start by taking a few deep, relaxing breaths, in through your nose and out through your mouth. Allow each exhalation to relax you more deeply. Once you feel completely relaxed, you are ready to begin.

Eleanor lost 34 cm (13½ in)!

'The weight I've lost (27 kg/60 lb) is exciting, but knowing that I have lost 17 cm (6½ in) from one thigh and 18 cm (7 in) from the other is totally amazing.

These thigh moves are so easy to do. They take only minutes to complete three times weekly, and they are totally effective! I can really "feel the burn". The exercises don't take much longer than the original *8 Minutes in the Morning*, but are totally targeted to work the entire thigh.

The People Solution has been KEY to my success, too! Communication with my friends (by e-mail, on the phone, at JorgeCruise.com, or in person) is what I *really* need, not food! One other thing... When I was a kid, one of the nicknames I was called was "Thunder Thighs". NOW, I'm working to have THINNER THIGHS!'

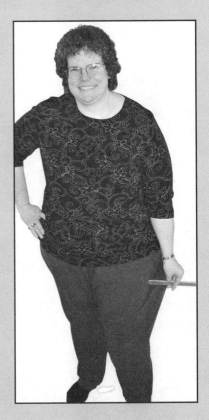

Eleanor was also featured on NBC's Ultimate Diet Challenge, where the Jorge Cruise® Plan was compared to five other leading national programmes. She ended up losing more weight than those on SlimFast®and Weight Watchers®. Congratulations, Eleanor!

seeing yourself clearly

Visualize yourself, standing in front of you. See your face and body. See your outfit and hairstyle. Notice how the person – you – standing in front of you feels right now. Become aware of any negative feelings – stress, anger, depression and so on. Feel love and compassion toward the 'you' in front of you, just as you would feel toward a child experiencing these same negative feelings. Allow the love you have stored up in your heart to expand and grow and fill up the 'you' standing in front of you. See yourself become filled with compassionate, loving energy. See yourself comforting and hugging the 'you' that you see in front of you. See yourself smile.

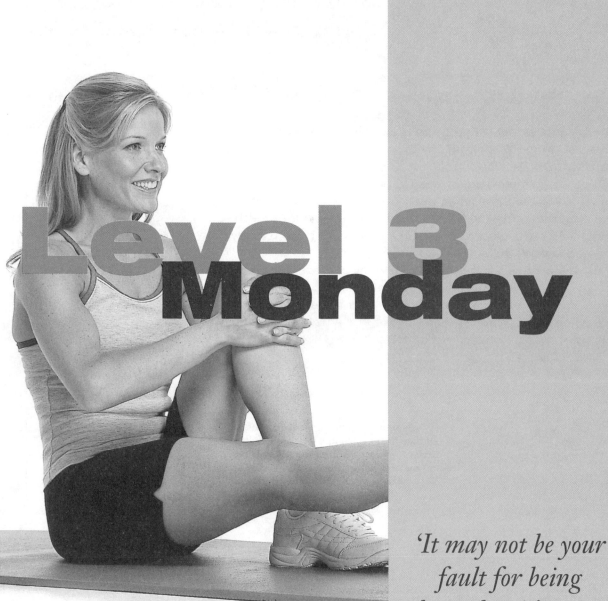

Level 3
Monday

'It may not be your fault for being down, but it's going to be your fault for not getting up.'

Steve Davis

jorge's power thought

You need protein to help build lean muscle, and fish is one of the best protein sources around. Besides quality protein, certain types of cold-water fatty fish contain a special type of fat called omega-3 fatty acids. These special fats have been shown to help reduce muscle soreness after a workout. They also help to boost your mood, turn down your appetite and give your skin a radiant glow.

What type of fish should you eat? I recommend salmon – it's very rich in omega-3 fatty acids. Organic or wild salmon is better than farmed salmon, which can have high levels of contaminants such as PCBs and mercury. Fresh tuna, mackerel and sardines are also good sources of omega-3 fatty acids.

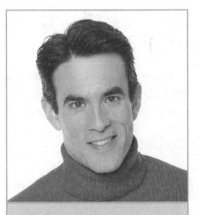

'The fatty acids in cold-water fish such as salmon are important for helping your muscles recover from your Cruise Moves.'

8 minute moves®
thighs day

MOVE 1: reclined pillow squeeze
inner thighs

a. Lie on your back with your knees bent and your feet on the floor. Place a thick, firm pillow between your thighs.

b. Exhale as you lift your hips, balancing your body weight on your upper back and feet. Squeeze the pillow between your thighs as if you were trying to squeeze the stuffing out of it. Hold for 40 to 60 seconds as you breathe normally. Release and proceed to Move 2.

a

b

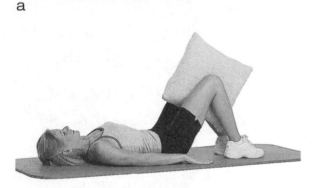
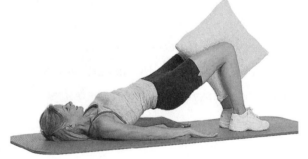

8-MINUTE LOG				
exercise	move 1	move 2	move 3	move 4
sets				
reps				

MOVE 2: doggie hold
outer thighs and hips

a. Kneel on your hands and knees. Make sure your hands are under your shoulders and your knees are under your hips.

b. Keeping your leg bent at a 90-degree angle, exhale as you lift your right leg out to the side (like a dog at a tree). Hold for 30 seconds. Lower and repeat with the other leg, then proceed to Move 3 on page 162.

a

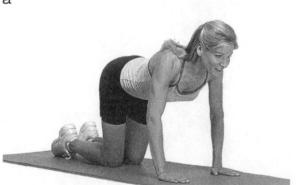

b

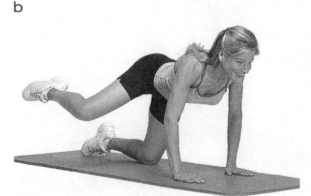

exercise sequence

1. warm up Jog or march on the spot for 1 minute.

2. cruise moves Do one 60-second repetition of each of your 4 Cruise Moves. Repeat this cycle and you will be done in 8 minutes.

3. cool down After your Cruise Moves, do these stretches (see page 74).

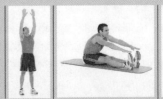

Sky-reaching pose | Hurdler's stretch | Cobra stretch

thighs day (cont'd)

MOVE 3: seated leg lift
fronts of the thighs

a. Sit on the floor with your left leg bent and your right leg extended. Wrap your hands around your left knee for support. Sit with your back long and straight. Try not to slouch.

b. Exhale as you lift your extended right leg as high as you can. Hold for 30 seconds while you breathe normally. Lower and repeat with the other leg, then proceed to Move 4.

a

b

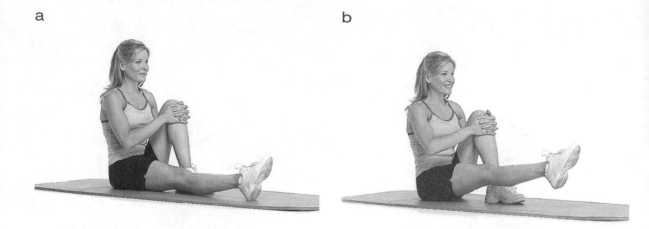

eat nutritionally, *not* emotionally®
visualization

Today you will use the power of your mind-body connection to fuel your motivation to stick to your Cruise Down Plate. During today's visualization, you will imagine a whole day's worth of your favourite healthy food choices. So close your eyes and take a few deep, relaxing breaths, in through your nose and out through your mouth. Allow each exhalation to bring you to a state of deep relaxation. Once you feel completely relaxed, you're ready to begin.

MOVE 4: kneeling leg lift
backs of the thighs and rear end

a. Kneel on the floor with your hands under your shoulders and your knees under your hips.

b. Exhale as you extend and lift your right leg slightly higher than your torso. Hold for 30 seconds. Release and repeat with your left leg, then return to Move 1 on page 160. Repeat Moves 1–4 once more and you're done.

a

b

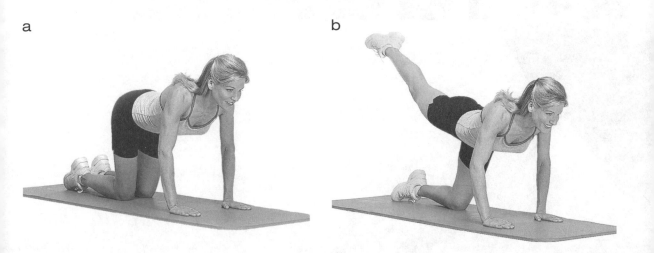

seeing healthy foods

You're heading to the kitchen to prepare yourself a wholesome breakfast. Will you be filling your Cruise Down Plate with scrambled egg whites, a piece of wholemeal toast with a little butter, and an orange?

Three hours later, it's time for a snack. Will you have some nuts? What about lunch? Will you join a friend for sushi and soup? Three hours later it's time

for another snack. What'll it be? A handful of raisins or maybe a yogurt? Three hours later, you've got a dinner date. Decide which veggies will fill your plate. What else will you have? And then of course, you have a special treat, possibly a square of chocolate. Remember, food is fuel and your body feels so great when you give it what it needs.

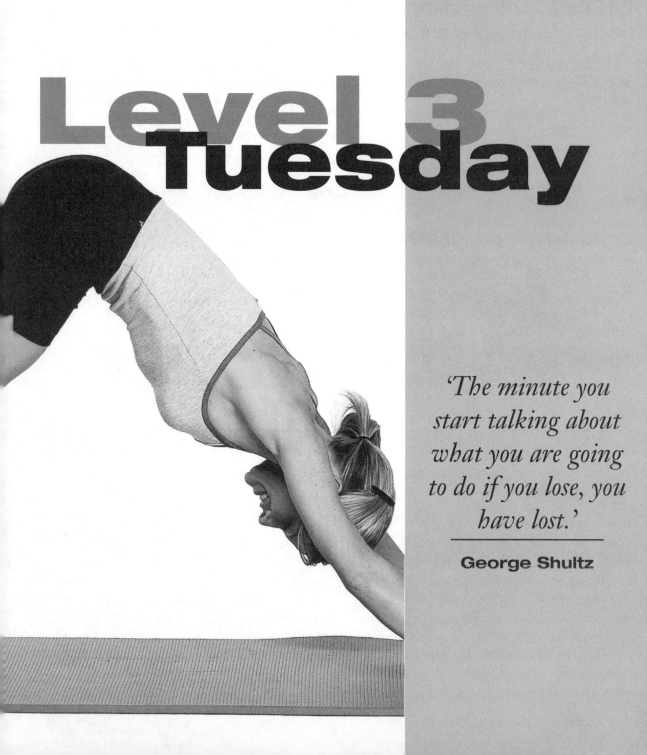

Level 3
Tuesday

'The minute you start talking about what you are going to do if you lose, you have lost.'

George Shultz

jorge's power thought

Have you ever watched a child eat? They eat a bite, squirm about as they chew it and, of course, play with their food. Plus, they always stop when they've had enough. Is there something we can learn here? You bet! Children listen to the instinctual cues that their bodies send them, so they stop when they're full. If you pay close attention while you eat, you'll notice that the pleasure you get from food tends to diminish as you continue to eat. This is a sign that your body has had enough, but many people eat so fast that they don't notice this signal. *Bring your inner child to the table.* Go ahead and have fun with your food when nobody's looking, and make it last. Make train tracks with your fork in your mashed potatoes; eat your sandwich crust first to make a funny shape. Your dinner will be a lot more fun and you'll probably eat a lot less.

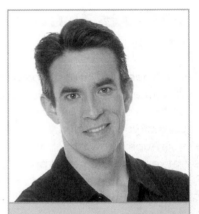

'The more slowly you eat and the more you chew your food, the more likely you'll stop eating before it's too late.'

8 minute moves®
upper-body day

MOVE 1: push-up
chest

a. Kneel with your palms on the floor under your chest. Extend one leg and then the other, so that your body weight is balanced on the balls of your feet and your palms. (You can do push-ups with your knees bent if you are not yet ready for standard push-ups.) Your fingers should be pointing forward and your toes pointing down.

b. Keep your back straight as you inhale, bend your elbows, and lower your torso towards the floor. Stop once your elbows are even with your shoulders. Exhale and push up to the starting position. Repeat for up to 1 minute, then proceed to Move 2.

a

b

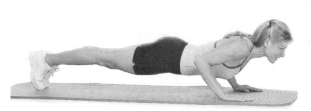

8-MINUTE LOG				
exercise	move 1	move 2	move 3	move 4
sets				
reps				

MOVE 2: yoga down dog
upper back

a. Kneel on all fours. Lower your hips to your heels and reach your palms as far forward as you can while still keeping your palms against the floor.

b. Exhale as you lift your buttocks toward the ceiling, bringing your body into a V shape. Press your palms into the floor as you lower your chest toward the floor and lift your tailbone toward the ceiling. Breathe normally as you hold for 1 minute. Return to the starting position, then proceed to Move 3 on page 168.

a

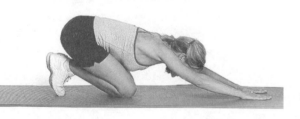

b

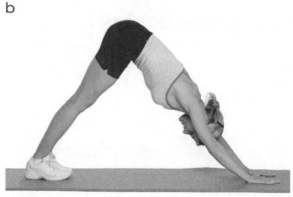

---

exercise sequence

1. warm up Jog or march on the spot for 1 minute.

2. cruise moves Do one 60-second repetition of each of your 4 Cruise Moves. Repeat this cycle and you will be done in 8 minutes.

3. cool down After your Cruise Moves, do these stretches (see page 74).

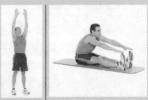

Sky-reaching pose | Hurdler's stretch | Cobra stretch

upper-body day (cont'd)

MOVE 3: low hover
triceps

a. From the down dog position, lower your hips until you're in a push-up position with your hands under your shoulders.

b. Slowly bend your elbows and lower your torso towards the floor, keeping your elbows close to your body. Stop 3–5 cm (1–2 in) above the floor. Hold and 'hover' for up to 60 seconds as you breathe normally. Release and proceed to Move 4.

a

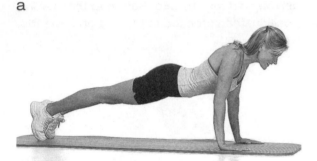

b

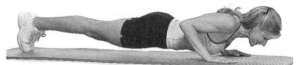

eat nutritionally, *not* emotionally® visualization

Today you will again use the power of visualization to help fuel healthy eating choices. Today you're going to prepare a delicious salad made with vegetables you've grown yourself in your very own garden. Today's visualization will make it possible!

Close your eyes and take a few relaxing breaths, in through your nose and out through your mouth. Allow each exhalation to bring you to a state of deep relaxation. Once you feel completely relaxed, you're ready to begin.

MOVE 4: 'show off my muscle' hold
biceps

a. Sit or stand. Firm your abdominals, lengthen and straighten your back and relax your shoulders. Raise your arms out to the sides, with your palms facing up. Curl your hands in loose fists toward your shoulders. Once in position, show off those muscles! Firm and flex your biceps (the muscles along the upper front of your arms) and hold for 60 seconds, breathing normally. Release, then return to Move 1 on page 166. Repeat Moves 1–4 once more and you're done.

a

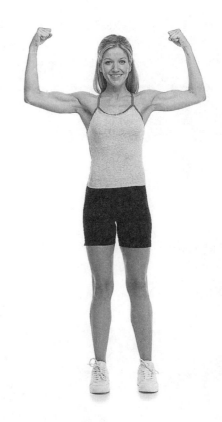

your inner garden

You've just returned from your local garden centre with everything you need to start your garden – soil, seeds or plants, shovel, hoe, watering can, and gloves. You slip on a pair of overalls, put on some sunscreen, and place a wide-brimmed hat on your head. Feel the sun warm your cheeks as you start hoeing the soil. Your arms are strong and firm. As you dig in the soil and plant each seed or plant, concentrate on how strong your body feels. You treat the garden with gentle care, giving it the nutrients it needs to grow! Picture how the garden will look in a few weeks and then in a month. Imagine the vegetables growing ripe and delicious.

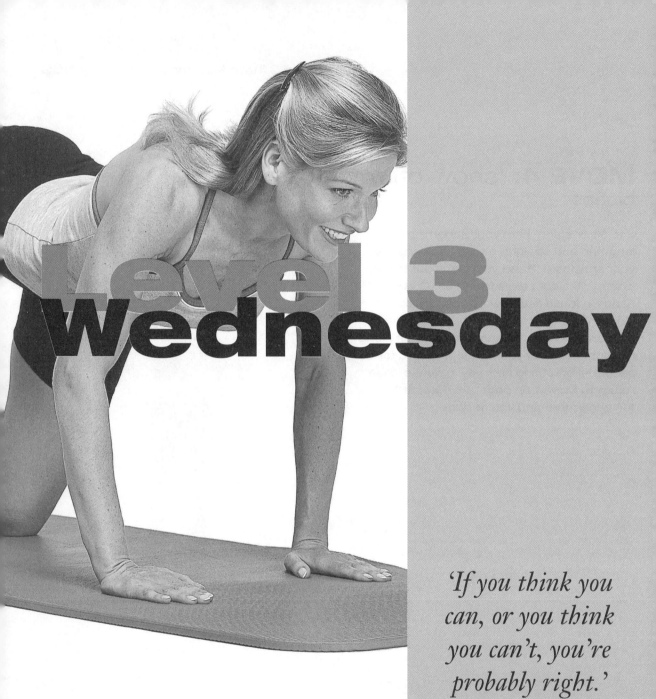

Level 3
Wednesday

'If you think you
can, or you think
you can't, you're
probably right.'

Mark Twain

jorge's power thought

One of the best ways to pamper yourself is with a massage. Whether you pay a professional or get a massage from a loved one, it has the same effect. The motion of the massage helps to increase circulation to your muscles as well as break up any knots or tense spots. This helps your muscles to recover from your Cruise Moves and prevents soreness.

But massage does even more. New research shows that your metabolism gets a boost when you get a massage. So, while you are relaxing on the table, you'll burn up some extra calories without lifting a finger! Also, there's nothing like the sensation of warm touch to help you relax and release all of your emotional worries. Indeed, regular massages are good for mind, body and soul. Treat yourself to one today. You've earned it!

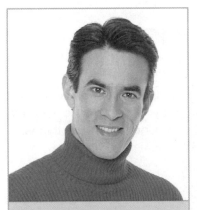

'Getting a massage is one of the best gifts you can give your body.'

8 minute moves®
thighs day

MOVE 1: reclined pillow squeeze
inner thighs

a. Lie on your back with your knees bent and your feet on the floor. Place a thick, firm pillow between your thighs.

b. Exhale as you lift your hips, balancing your body weight on your upper back and feet. Squeeze the pillow between your thighs as if you were trying to squeeze the stuffing out of it. Hold for 40 to 60 seconds as you breathe normally. Release and proceed to Move 2.

a

b

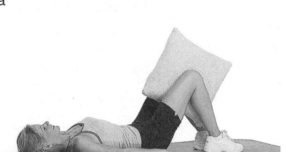
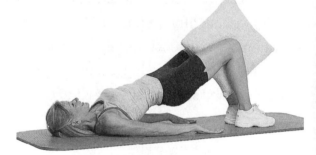

8-MINUTE LOG				
exercise	move 1	move 2	move 3	move 4
sets				
reps				

MOVE 2: doggie hold
outer thighs and hips

a. Kneel on your hands and knees. Make sure your hands are under your shoulders and your knees are under your hips.

b. Keeping your leg bent at a 90-degree angle, exhale as you lift your right leg out to the side (like a dog at a tree). Hold for 30 seconds. Lower and repeat with the other leg, then proceed to Move 3 on page 174.

a

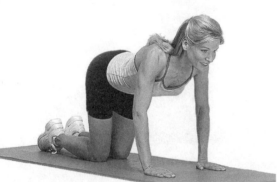

b

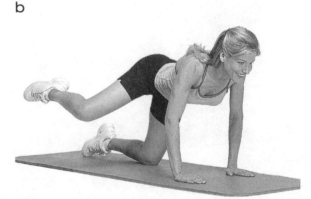

exercise sequence

1. warm up Jog or march on the spot for 1 minute.

2. cruise moves Do one 60-second repetition of each of your 4 Cruise Moves. Repeat this cycle and you will be done in 8 minutes.

3. cool down After your Cruise Moves, do these stretches (see page 74).

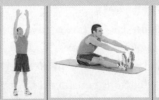

Sky-reaching pose | Hurdler's stretch | Cobra stretch

thighs day (cont'd)

MOVE 3: seated leg lift
fronts of the thighs

a. Sit on the floor with your left leg bent and your right leg extended. Wrap your hands around your left knee for support. Sit with your back long and straight. Try not to slouch.

b. Exhale as you lift your extended right leg as high as you can. Hold for 30 seconds while you breathe normally. Lower and repeat with the other leg, then proceed to Move 4.

a

b

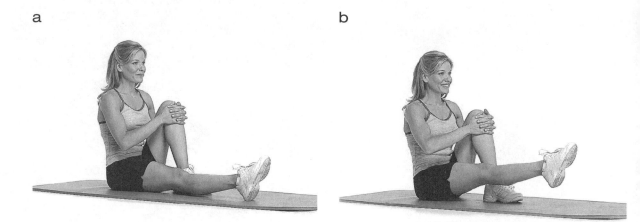

eat nutritionally, *not* emotionally® visualization

Today you will again use the power of visualization to help fuel healthy eating choices. Today is your best friend's birthday and you've invited her over for a healthy and delicious gourmet dinner. Are you ready to get cooking? Close your eyes and take a few relaxing breaths, in through your nose and out through your mouth. Allow each exhalation to bring you to a state of deep relaxation. Once you feel completely relaxed, you're ready to begin.

MOVE 4: kneeling leg lift
backs of the thighs and rear end

a. Kneel on the floor with your hands under your shoulders and your knees under your hips.

b. Exhale as you extend and lift your right leg slightly higher than your torso. Hold for 30 seconds. Release and repeat with your left leg, then return to Move 1 on page 172. Repeat Moves 1–4 once more and you're done.

a

b

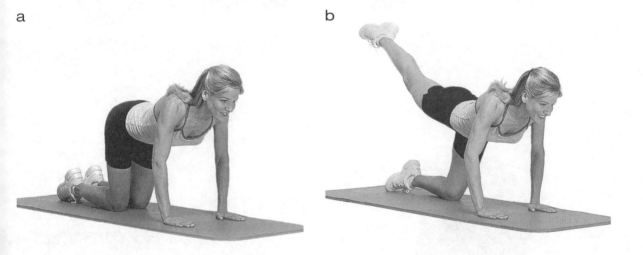

a gourmet meal

You carefully planned the menu earlier in the week and purchased everything you need. You hear the doorbell ring just as you finish chopping the last few veggies for the salad. See yourself open the door and greet your friend with a big birthday hug. You lead her to the dining table, which you've set with your best dishes. See yourself serving each yummy dish. Enjoy each bite and stop eating when you're satisfied, not overly full.

When dinner is cleared, you dim the lights and bring out the cake. She blows out the candles and you each savour a slice. She gives you a big hug and says, 'Thank you so much! This really made me feel special. You are a great friend'.

Level 3
Thursday

'The pessimist sees the difficulty in every opportunity; the optimist, the opportunity in every difficulty.'

L. P. Jacks

jorge's power thought

I'm sure you've noticed how much better you feel throughout the day after you do your Cruise Moves in the morning. That's not the half of it. Psychologists and exercise physiologists have found that exercise may actually work as well as drugs for treating depression.

A study done at Duke University in the US recently tested this theory. They recruited 156 men and women age 50 and older who suffered from major depression. One group walked or jogged for 30 minutes 3 days a week, while another group took an antidepressant. At the end of 4 months, both groups had improved dramatically. When the researchers checked back 6 months later to see how the people were faring on their own, 38 per cent of the antidepressant group had fallen back into depression, but only 8 per cent of the exercise group saw their symptoms return.

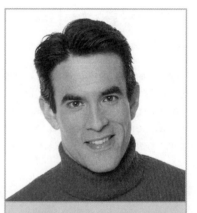

'Your Cruise Moves can help lift your spirits all day long – making you literally start the day on the right foot.'

8 minute moves®
torso and calves day

MOVE 1: half-forward bend
belly

a. Stand with your feet under your hips and your knees slightly bent. Inhale as you raise your arms out to the sides and up overhead. Lengthen your spine and reach the crown of your head toward the ceiling.

b. Exhale as you bend forward from the hips, reaching through your fingertips. Stop once your torso and legs form a 90-degree angle. Reach back through your tailbone and forward through your fingertips and the crown of your head. Hold for up to 60 seconds, breathing normally. Inhale and return to the starting position, then proceed to Move 2.

a

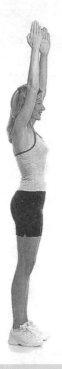

b

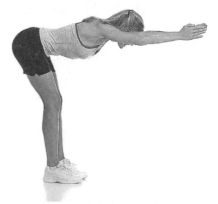

8-MINUTE LOG				
exercise	move 1	move 2	move 3	move 4
sets				
reps				

MOVE 2: balancing stick
lower back

a. Stand with your feet under your hips and your hands at your sides. Step forward with your right foot, keeping both legs extended. Inhale as you raise your arms overhead.

b. Exhale as you bend forward from the hips and simultaneously raise your extended left leg behind until your left leg, torso and arms are parallel with the floor. Hold for up to 30 seconds, breathing normally. Release, return to the starting position, and repeat with the other leg. Then proceed to Move 3 on page 180.

a

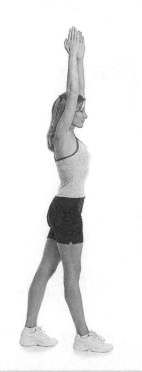

b

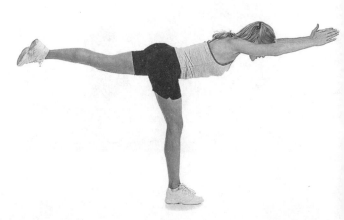

exercise sequence

1. warm up Jog or march on the spot for 1 minute.

2. cruise moves Do one 60-second repetition of each of your 4 Cruise Moves. Repeat this cycle and you will be done in 8 minutes.

3. cool down After your Cruise Moves, do these stretches (see page 74).

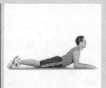

Sky-reaching pose | Hurdler's stretch | Cobra stretch

torso and calves day (cont'd)

MOVE 3: half-handstand
shoulders

a. Kneel with your back to a wall, both feet against the wall. Place your hands under your chest.

b. Lift one leg and place the ball of the foot against the wall. Do the same with the other foot and then walk your feet up the wall until you can straighten your arms, legs and back. Your torso should be perpendicular to the floor. Hold for up to 60 seconds. Release, then proceed to Move 4. *Note:* If this move is difficult for you, do it with your feet on the ground.

a

b

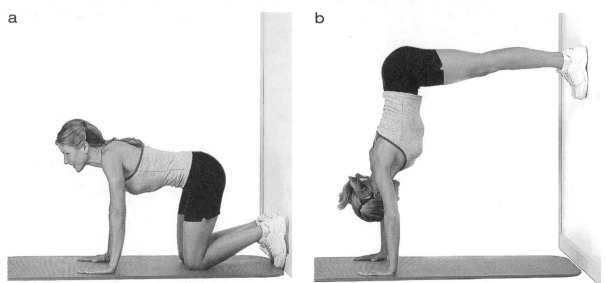

eat nutritionally, *not* emotionally®
visualization

Today you will strengthen your motivation to stick with the Cruise Down Plate by visualizing yourself in the future. You will envision a day after you've reached your goal, a day when your hips and thighs are slimmer than you've ever dreamed! Today, you're preparing for a very special date. So, first

relax by closing your eyes and taking a few deep, relaxing breaths, in through your nose and out through your mouth. Allow each exhalation to bring you to a state of deep relaxation. Once you feel completely relaxed, you're ready to begin.

MOVE 4: yoga down dog with leg raise
calves

a. Kneel on all fours. Lower your hips to your heels and reach your palms as far forward as you can while still keeping your palms against the floor.

b. Exhale as you lift your buttocks toward the ceiling, bringing your body into a V shape. Press your palms into the floor as you lower your chest toward the floor and lift your tailbone toward the ceiling.

c. Rise onto the balls of your feet. Shift your body weight onto your right foot. Lift your extended left leg as high as possible. Hold for 30 seconds. Switch legs and repeat, then return to Move 1 on page 178. Repeat Moves 1–4 once more and you're done.

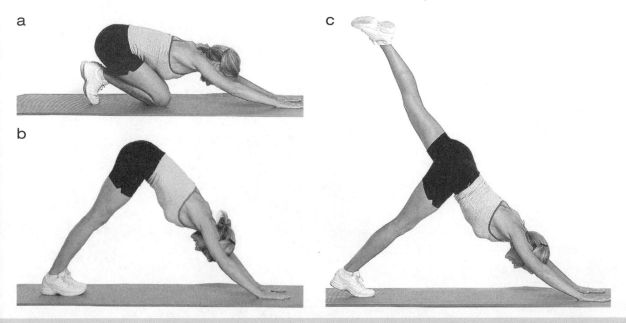

a

b

c

your first date

See yourself getting ready for your date. Who will be your date for the evening? How do you prepare for your date? See yourself taking a hot bubble bath or splurging on a manicure and facial. Then, pick out a beautiful outfit from the back of your wardrobe, one that you've always loved but refused to wear because of your hips and thighs. Maybe it has a slit high up on the leg. Put it on. See how great your legs look in this outfit! Look in the mirror and twirl around and smile at how slim and healthy you look.

Hear the doorbell ring. Open the door and see your date. Hear your date comment on how lovely you look. What does your date say and how does it make you feel?

Level 3
Friday

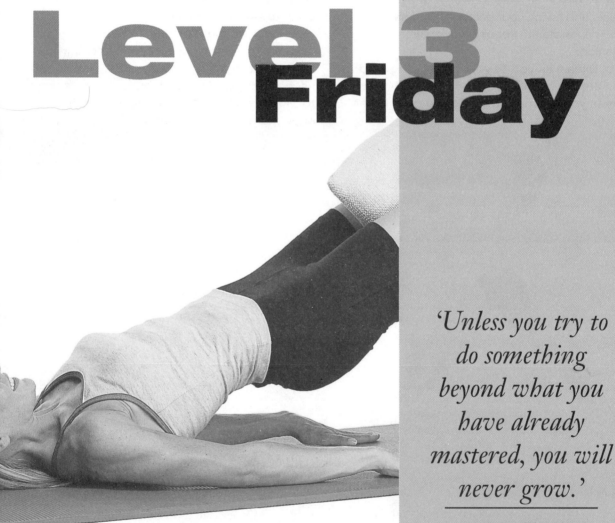

'Unless you try to do something beyond what you have already mastered, you will never grow.'

Ralph Waldo Emerson

jorge's power thought

Even if you eat a healthy diet that is rich in vegetables and whole grains, you may still be deficient in many important nutrients. In fact, the *Journal of the American Medical Association* recently reported that 'most people do not consume an optimal amount of all vitamins by diet alone' and that 'all adults should take one multivitamin daily'.

A multivitamin provides extra insurance that you get all of the vitamins and minerals you need, particularly on those extra busy days when you don't eat as well as you should. Make sure your multivitamin contains roughly 100 per cent of the recommended daily intake for most vitamins and minerals. Note that because calcium is a very bulky mineral, most multivitamins only contain a small amount of it. If you have trouble swallowing pills and capsules, that's no excuse to skip your multi. There are plenty of liquid multivitamins on the market.

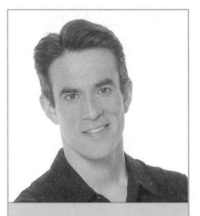

'A multivitamin provides extra insurance that you get all of the vitamins and minerals you need.'

8 minute moves®
thighs day

MOVE 1: reclined pillow squeeze
inner thighs

a. Lie on your back with your knees bent and your feet on the floor. Place a thick, firm pillow between your thighs.

b. Exhale as you lift your hips, balancing your body weight on your upper back and feet. Squeeze the pillow between your thighs as if you were trying to squeeze the stuffing out of it. Hold for 40 to 60 seconds as you breathe normally. Release and proceed to Move 2.

a

b

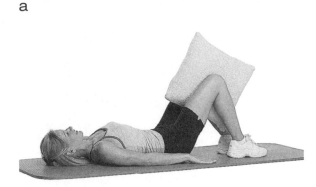

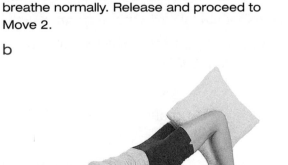

8-MINUTE LOG				
exercise	move 1	move 2	move 3	move 4
sets				
reps				

MOVE 2: doggie hold
outer thighs and hips

a. Kneel on your hands and knees. Make sure your hands are under your shoulders and your knees are under your hips.

b. Keeping your leg bent at a 90-degree angle, exhale as you lift your right leg out to the side (like a dog at a tree). Hold for 30 seconds. Lower and repeat with the other leg, then proceed to Move 3 on page 186.

a

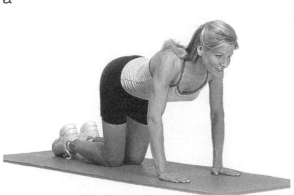

b

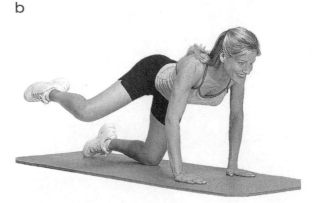

exercise sequence

1. warm up Jog or march on the spot for 1 minute.

2. cruise moves Do one 60-second repetition of each of your 4 Cruise Moves. Repeat this cycle and you will be done in 8 minutes.

3. cool down After your Cruise Moves, do these stretches (see page 74).

Sky-reaching pose | Hurdler's stretch | Cobra stretch

thighs day (cont'd)

MOVE 3: seated leg lift
fronts of the thighs

a. Sit on the floor with your left leg bent and your right leg extended. Wrap your hands around your left knee for support. Sit with your back long and straight. Try not to slouch.

b. Exhale as you lift your extended right leg as high as you can. Hold for 30 seconds while you breathe normally. Lower and repeat with the other leg, then proceed to Move 4.

a

b

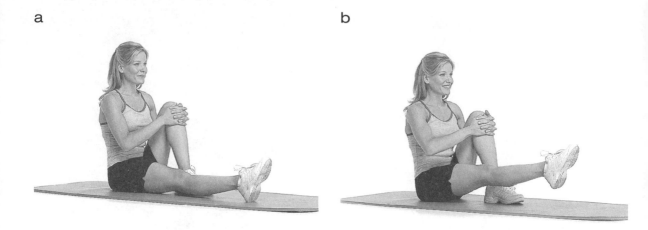

eat nutritionally, *not* emotionally® visualization

Today we will nurture your inner motivation with a very special visualization exercise. During today's visualization, you will be reunited with an old friend who hasn't seen you for many years. So, close your eyes and take a few relaxing breaths, in through your nose and out through your mouth. Allow each exhalation to bring you to a state of deep relaxation. Once you feel completely relaxed, you're ready to begin.

MOVE 4: kneeling leg lift
backs of the thighs and rear end

a. Kneel on the floor with your hands under your shoulders and your knees under your hips.

b. Exhale as you extend and lift your right leg slightly higher than your torso. Hold for 30 seconds. Release and repeat with your left leg, then return to Move 1 on page 184. Repeat Moves 1–4 once more and you're done.

a

b

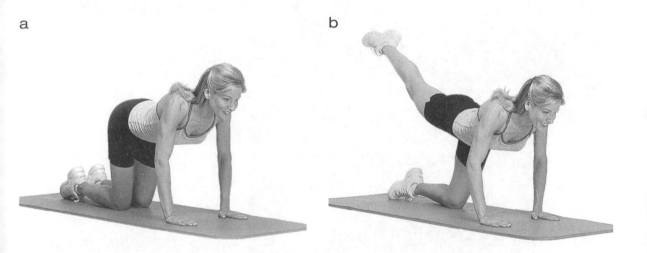

seeing an old friend

See yourself pulling into the car park at the airport to pick up your friend. Take a quick look in the rearview mirror and smile at your reflection. You look healthier, happier and younger than you have in years! You have only a few minutes until your friend's flight is due at the gate, so you quickly head to the stairs and mount them two at a time. Feel how agile and strong your body feels as you quickly climb each staircase. You make it just in time to see your friend approach. She smiles politely, says, 'Excuse me,' and brushes past you. She doesn't recognize you! You call her name and say, 'It's me!' Your friend turns around stunned and says, 'You look incredible! What have you done?' You smile radiantly.

Level 3
Saturday

'Hard work won't guarantee you a thing, but without it, you don't stand a chance.'

Patrick Riley

jorge's power thought

Eggs have gained a bad reputation over the last few decades because health experts thought that eggs raised blood cholesterol levels. In the last few years, numerous health organizations have been vindicating eggs' reputation.

The key is just to use the whites of the eggs. That's where all the protein is that your muscles need in order to grow. The saturated fat in an egg is in the yolk, so I suggest you just eat the protein-rich egg white or try an egg substitute.

Start your day right by making an egg white omelette with lots of veggies. One of my favourite omelettes is made with chopped spinach, chopped peppers, chopped cooked soya sausage, chopped tomatoes and a carton of egg substitute.

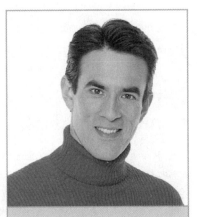

'Some egg substitutes are pasteurized, meaning they're safe to eat without cooking. I use them as the base in smoothies to add more appetite-suppressing protein.'

stretches
day off from cruise moves

Today is your day off from your Cruise Moves. To accelerate your results, I suggest that you spend 8 minutes this morning stretching and lengthening your muscles.

STRETCH 1: kneeling thigh stretch
fronts of the thighs

a. Kneel on your hands and knees with your back to a wall. Lift your left knee, placing your left shin and foot against the wall.

b. Lift your right knee, bringing your right foot onto the floor into a modified lunge position.

c. To increase the stretch, lift your torso, placing your hands on your right thigh. The closer you bring your back toward the wall, the more intense the stretch will become. Hold for 30 seconds, breathing normally. Release and then repeat with the other leg. Then proceed to Stretch 2.

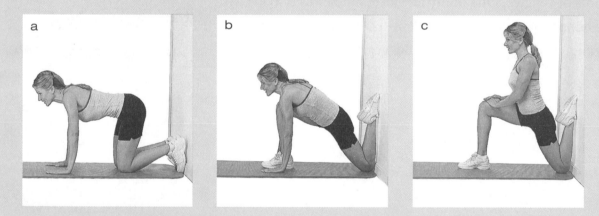

eat nutritionally, *not* emotionally®
visualization

Sometimes during the course of a day, we tend to focus only on the negative. We forget all of the good things. When we focus only on the negative, we allow negative emotions such as sadness, guilt and anger to build out of proportion to reality.

And when that happens, we run to the refrigerator!

Today's visualization will help you keep negative emotions in check with reality. Start by taking a few deep, relaxing breaths. Once you feel completely relaxed, you are ready to begin.

STRETCH 2: pigeon yoga stretch
outer thighs and hips

a. Start on all fours with your hands under your chest and your knees under your hips. Lift your left knee and draw it as far forward between your arms as possible. Externally rotate your left thigh, resting your outer left thigh near your left hand and your left heel near your right hip, with the toes pointing to the right. Reach back with your right leg, extending it and placing the top of your right foot on the floor. Keep the sides of your hips even and parallel to the floor.

b. To increase the stretch, reach forward with your hands, resting your torso on your left inner thigh. Hold for 30 seconds, breathing normally. Release and switch legs, then proceed to Stretch 3 on page 192.

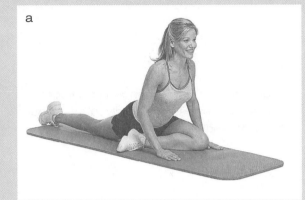

cultivating gratitude

Visualize your entire day yesterday. Call to mind every good thing that happened during the entire 24-hour period. Remember every compliment. Remember the traffic lights that were green instead of red. Remember the luck of finding the prime parking space. Recall any instances when someone treated you kindly. Recall any simple pleasures that you experienced, such as the smell of blooming spring flowers or the sight of a rare bird. Take a few more moments to reflect on every good thing that took place yesterday. As you do so, feel your gratitude growing and growing.

stretches
day off from cruise moves (cont'd)

STRETCH 3: seated forward bend
backs of the thighs

a. Sit with your legs extended and your hands at your sides. Inhale as you raise your arms overhead.

b. Exhale as you bend forward, keeping your spine long and straight. Lower your arms to your ankles or shins. Hold and breathe normally for 60 seconds, then release and proceed to Stretch 4.

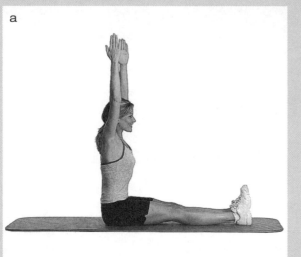

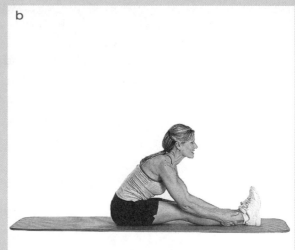

STRETCH 4: butterfly stretch
inner thighs

a. Sit on the floor. Bend your legs and bring the outer edges of your feet together. Release your knees out to the sides. Grasp your ankles with your hands.

b. Exhale as you lean forward from the hips. Try to keep your spine long and straight. Hold for 60 seconds as you breathe normally. Inhale and rise to the starting position, then return to Stretch 1 on page 190. Repeat Stretches 1–4 once more and you're done.

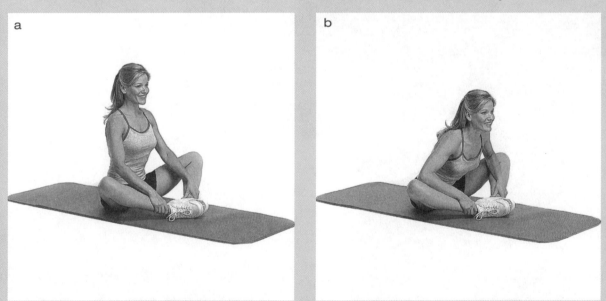

Level 3
Sunday

'Look at a day when you are supremely satisfied at the end. It's not a day when you lounge around doing nothing. It's when you've had everything to do, and you've done it.'

Margaret Thatcher

jorge's power thought

Water is so important to your success. Your body is made up of 75 per cent water. Your body needs water to create a fluid blood volume. When you become dehydrated, your blood becomes viscous and sticky, making it harder for your heart to pump it through your body. This raises your heart rate, making you feel overly tired during simple movements like your Cruise Moves. Worse, your brain can't distinguish between dehydration and starvation, and responds to both by emitting hunger signals. This means that even though your body is not in need of food, you will feel fatigued, restless and hungry, when all you really need is a tall glass of water. So instead of getting mixed signals from your body, just give it what it needs: lots of water.

I like to drink a tall glass of water first thing in the morning, right before I do my Cruise Moves. I find that it helps energize me.

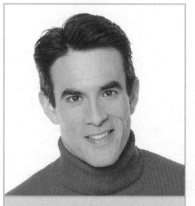

'Whenever you feel tired, drink a glass of water. You may really only be dehydrated.'

capture your progress
day off from cruise moves

Today is your day off. Take a moment to relish your progress. Grab a pen and answer the following questions.

1. What is your current weight?

_____

2. What was your original weight?

_____

3. What is your waist circumference?

_____

4. What was your original waist circumference?

_____

5. What have you done well this week? What are you most proud of?

_____

_____

_____

_____

_____

6. What could you improve next week?

_____

_____

_____

_____

_____

eat nutritionally, *not* emotionally®
visualization

Sometimes our zeal to control situations is what gets us into trouble emotionally. Today's visualization will help you set aside your problems, allowing yourself to love your life, no matter how it presents itself to you. Start by taking a few moments to relax.

Take a few deep breaths, in through your nose and out through your mouth, using your exhalations to bring you to a deeper and deeper state of relaxation. Once you feel deeply relaxed, you are ready to begin.

bonnie lost 10 cm (4 in) from her thighs!

'Jorge's programme has been great for me, and I am so proud of what I have accomplished. I've lost a total of 15 kg (33 lb). My thighs have firmed and my bottom has lifted. For the first time in many, many years I bought a pair of shorts. I also recently had fun trying on swimsuits. Clothes shopping is now an awesome experience. I even recently fit into a pair of hipster jeans. I was a kid when I last wore that style of jeans, and now I am finally donning them again and getting so many compliments.

The results are fantastic. My thighs have always been a trouble zone for me, and now I have the tools to zap them! Because the programme is so simple and needs so little equipment, it's easy to make it a priority in my life.

I now feel that I have control over eating and my life. I am choosing to live a healthy lifestyle. This programme has added years to my life as well as taken years off my appearance. I look and feel so much younger than the day I started the programme.'

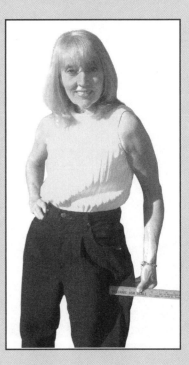

Bonnie went from a size 14 to a size 8.

letting go

Ponder a problem that you are having. Perhaps you are experiencing conflict with your children or maybe you worry about your spouse's frequent late nights at work. Pick just one situation that tends to make you feel at the end of your tether – one to which you see no active solution. Imagine that you are holding your problem in the palms of your hands. Imagine a hope chest in the room. Carry your problem over to the hope chest. Open the lid and carefully place your problem in the bottom of the chest for safekeeping. Close the lid and walk away. Notice how free you feel when you relieve yourself of the need to control or worry about a problem that you can't solve!

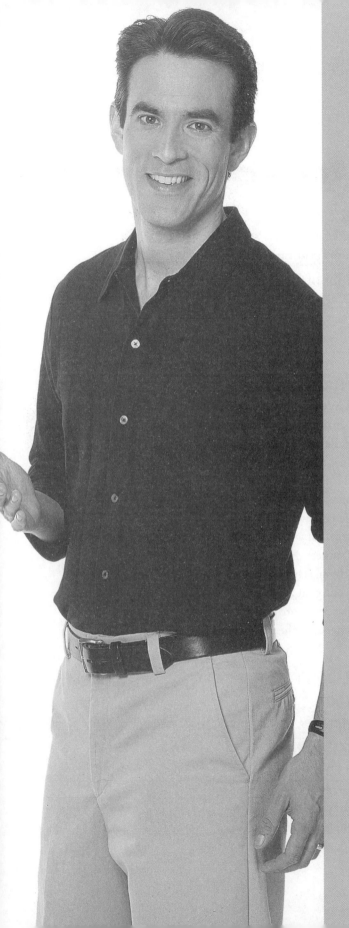

Bonus Chapter

Get Longer, Leaner Legs <u>Even</u> Faster

three ways to accelerate your results

My Cruise Moves and eating plan will help you build long, sleek muscles that will help burn 1 kg (2 lb) of fat a week. You'll consistently shrink the size of your hips and thighs by boosting your metabolism.

So far, I've provided you with a simple 2-step process for shrinking the size of your hips and thighs. Your first step – 8 minutes of Cruise Moves – helped you to build the muscle needed to burn the fat. Your second step – Eat Nutritionally, *Not* Emotionally – helped to further support lean muscle growth and avoid emotional eating.

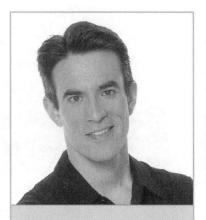

'No matter when you do it, it's best to stretch when your muscles are warm.'

That's all you need to see results. However, I know some of you are anxious to see results even faster. I know some of you want slimmer hips and thighs *yesterday*. That's where this bonus chapter comes in. This chapter will provide you with some additional secrets that will help accelerate your success. Follow the tips in this bonus chapter and you will meet your goal more quickly. You'll also create more energy and feel better from head to toe.

your '8 minute' edge

The three bonus tips in this chapter will help you to:

• Elongate your leg muscles

• Reduce the appearance of cellulite

• Help prevent varicose veins

• Accelerate your results

lengthen your muscles with regular stretching

In chapter 3, I suggested you use your 8 minutes of free time on Saturdays to your advantage by doing a simple, 8-minute stretching routine. And in your programme in chapter 5, you found some of my favourite stretches for the hips and thighs.

I'm a firm believer in the power of stretching, particularly when it comes to slimming the hips and thighs area. I've seen first-hand how a regular stretching routine helped my sister, Marta, create longer, leaner, sexier legs. I've also seen the results over and over in my clients.

And there's solid science to back up the powers of stretching. I've already told you that a stretching routine will help to lengthen your muscles. Regular stretching also helps improve circulation, which is important in helping your muscles to recover from your weekly Cruise Moves sessions. Also, stretching improves the health of your connective tissue, helping to prevent those little pockets of fat from bulging through and creating cellulite. Finally, stretching helps to improve your range of motion and flexibility, which, in turn,

help keep your muscles healthy.

Each Saturday in chapter 5, I suggested four 8-minute stretches for you to try. To accelerate your results even more, consider doing my suggested stretching routines every day or every other day. No matter when you do it, it's best to stretch when your muscles are warm. So do these stretches *after* your Cruise Moves, not before. If you don't have more than 8 minutes in the morning, you can also complete your stretching routine just before bedtime, when your muscles are already warm and pliable from moving around all day. In addition to accelerating your results, you'll also help to ready your body and mind for sleep. Many of my clients tell me that a short, pre-bedtime stretching routine helps them to fall asleep faster and sleep more deeply.

When you stretch, always exhale as you move your body into the stretch. Then hold the stretch for 30 to 60 seconds as you breathe normally. Research

has shown that 30 seconds is the minimum amount of time needed for a muscle to lengthen. If you hold the stretch for a shorter amount of time, you won't see results.

Try not to bounce while you stretch, as this can lead to injury. Also, if you feel especially tight in a particular muscle, it sometimes helps to visualize exhaling your breath through the tight muscle. This simple visualization helps coax your muscle to release, allowing you to stretch a bit longer.

improve circulation with regular massage

I often suggest that my clients reward themselves whenever they reach a goal. Some will reward themselves with a new outfit. Others reward themselves by taking a warm, luxurious bath. And some reward themselves with a professional massage.

Don't forget to stretch

Remember to do your stretches during each week of your *8 Minutes in the Morning for Lean Hips and Thin Thighs* programme! Your stretches for Level 1 are found on pages 110–113, your stretches for Level 2 are found on pages 150–53, and your stretches for Level 3 are found on pages 190–93. Remember, it's so important to stretch during this programme – it will help you create long, sleek hip and thigh muscles, and will let you see those sexy muscles even *faster*!

If you reward yourself with a professional massage, you'll reap some unexpected bonuses. Massage can do much more than help you to relax and feel pampered. Like stretching, massage also can help lengthen your muscles, creating a longer, leaner appearance. Massage also increases circulation to your muscles, helping them to recover faster from your Cruise Moves.

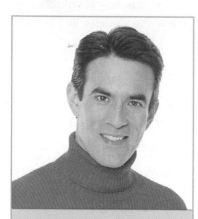

'Massage increases circulation to your muscles, helping them to recover faster.'

And new research shows that massage can also boost your metabolism. No other form of pampering gives you so much return on so little effort!

There are many different types of massage. Swedish massage, one of the most popular types offered at spas, involves long, light, relaxing strokes. If you're looking for a deeper touch, consider sports, deep muscle, or neuromuscular massage. In those types of massage, the therapist will dig his or her fingers, fists and elbows deep into your muscles. This helps to break up knots, but also results in some discomfort during the massage.

I often encourage my married clients to do a massage course with their partner. Not only does this help you bond and grow closer, it also provides a convenient and affordable way to reap the benefits of massage at home. Here are a few tips for coupling up:

Use cream or some other type of lubricant. This will allow your hands to glide and prevent you from chaffing each other's skin or accidentally yanking out fine body hairs.

Trim your nails. This will prevent accidental pinching and scratching.

Use firm, long strokes. For example, to massage the back of your partner's thigh, place the palm of your hand firmly against his or her thigh and then smoothly move your hand up his or her leg without stopping.

Start with your palms. Use the palms of your hands first. This will help warm up your partner's muscles. Then after a few long, even strokes with your palms, you can provide deeper and more specific pressure with your thumbs.

Communicate. Know that everyone's pain threshold is a little different. You might like very deep pressure, whereas your partner may desire a much lighter touch. As you massage one another, communicate with each other. There's a fine line between 'sore but good' and 'painful'. Make sure your partner knows where that line is. If you gently prompt your partner when to go deeper and when to back off, you'll enjoy your massage much more.

reverse gravity to reduce swelling

Your heart has no trouble pumping blood down your legs and to your feet. That's because gravity lends a helping hand. However, once blood gets to your feet, it must make its way back up your legs, against the pull of gravity, and this is where things can go awry.

The force of gravity is one of the main culprits of varicose veins. As blood tries to make its way back up your legs, gravity pulls it downward. If your heart doesn't beat strongly enough or the tiny muscles in your veins fail to effectively push blood upward, it can pool backward, enlarging the size of your veins.

You can do something about this and it's actually a very simple remedy. Every day after work or just before bed, lie on your back and elevate your legs up a wall, as shown, right.

In addition to helping to prevent varicose veins, elevating your legs will help move swelling out of your legs and feet. This will help reduce the appearance

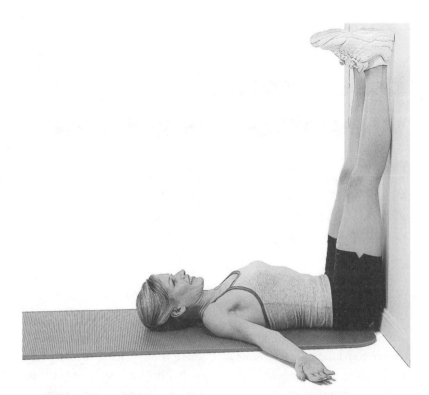

Legs Up the Wall Pose
Elevating your legs helps increase circulation, reduce swelling and prevent varicose veins.

of cellulite and give your thighs a smoother, sleeker appearance.

It also *feels* really good, particularly if your legs or feet are sore or tired. Make sure to do it any day you spend a lot of time on your feet. Your body will thank you!

become a weight-loss star

Here's a motivational incentive to keep you going. After you reach your goal weight, send me your weight-loss success story with before and after pictures and you may be selected for special recognition.

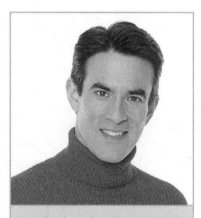

Plus, if you are selected, I might feature you during my television appearances, in my magazine columns, on my website, or in upcoming books. You'll become a weight-loss star. Each year, I host a red rose ceremony in San Diego, recognizing my most inspirational and successful clients. With help from my staff, we pick VIPs, who are introduced at this ceremony in an auditorium filled with Jorge Cruise clients. We will capture the event on camera so I can share your amazing success story with others. So, are you ready to become an inspirational role model to millions?

how to apply

Visit www.jorgecruise.com, write your story and send it, along with your 'before' and 'after' photos, to the address listed on the website.

Good luck and best wishes!

'Putting your body first gives you the health and energy you need to live your life to its fullest.'

the synergy pages

additional jorge cruise tools

Ready for more? Check out these synergistic ways to take the Jorge Cruise weight-control plan to the next level.

jorgecruise.com: the No. 1 online weight-control club for busy people

Staying motivated can get complicated sometimes. It can be tough tackling everything on your own. As one of my online clients you will have direct access to me and my LIVE coaches to ensure you lose 1 kg (2 lb) a week. Having this kind of support can be the difference between reaching the finish line and running on the spot.

top 6 reasons to join:

1. Accountability: get daily encouragement directly from me.

2. Accelerate Results: experience daily LIVE coaching from my personally trained mentors to help maximize your weight loss.

3. End Self-Sabotage: join daily virtual conversations posted by my other clients who have overcome emotional eating.

4. Find Buddies: 24/7 motivation and support in our Empowerment Circle.

5. Exclusive Tools: chart your weight loss with our specialized online tools.

6. The Latest Secrets: attend live auditoriums with me and all other members too!

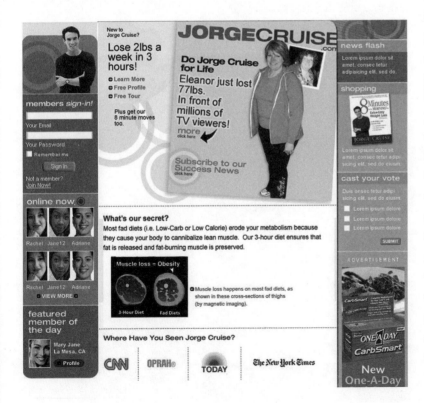

Joining our club is like joining a family.

the book series

Build your Jorge Cruise book collection and get all of my secrets to further help you lose up to 1 kg (2 lb) a week in just 8 minutes! The current full collection includes:

- *8 Minutes in the Morning*
- *8 Minutes in the Morning for Maximum Weight Loss*
- *8 Minutes in the Morning for a Flat Belly*
- *8 Minutes in the Morning for Lean Hips and Thin Thighs*
- *3-Hour Diet*™ (to be published 2005)

Visit www.jorgecruise.com for full details.

about the author

Jorge Cruise: The World's No. 1 Online Weight-Control Specialist

'Time is your most precious commodity… Don't waste it.'

Jorge Cruise

Jorge Cruise personally struggled with weight as a child and young man. Today he is recognized as America's leading weight-loss expert for busy people. He is the No. 1 *New York Times* bestselling author of *8 Minutes in the Morning*®, published in 14 languages, and the author of the forthcoming 3-Hour Diet™. Jorge has also coached over 3 million online clients at JorgeCruise.com and is the exclusive weight loss coach for AOL's 23 million subscribers. Each Sunday his *USA Weekend* column is read by more than 50 million readers in 600 newspapers. Jorge is also the 'Slimming Coach' columnist for the American magazine *First for Woman*, with over 3 million readers each month. In the US, he has appeared on *Oprah*, CNN, *Good Morning America*, *The Today Show*, *Dateline NBC* and *The View* with Barbara Walters. In the UK, he has appeared on GMTV and featured in *Top Santé, Slimming, Woman's Own, The Times, The Daily Mirror* and *The Independent on Sunday*.

Jorge lives in San Diego, California, with his wife and son. Visit JorgeCruise.com for details of his free personal coaching contest.

Utilizing the knowledge and credentials that he has gained from the University of California, San Diego (UCSD); Dartmouth College; the Cooper Institute for Aerobics Research; the American College of Sports Medicine (ACSM) and the American Council on Exercise (ACE), Jorge is dedicated to helping busy people lose weight without fad dieting.

OTHER RODALE BOOKS
AVAILABLE FROM PAN MACMILLAN

1-4050-2101-2	8 Minutes in the Morning	*Jorge Cruise*	£12.99
1-4050-4180-3	8 Minutes in the Morning for Maximum Weight Loss	*Jorge Cruise*	£12.99
1-4050-3284-7	Anti-Ageing Prescriptions	*Dr James A. Duke*	£14.99
1-4050-4179-X	Fit Not Fat at 40+	*The Editors of* Prevention	£12.99
1-4050-3335-5	Picture Perfect Weight Loss	*Dr Howard Shapiro*	£14.99
1-4050-6717-9	The South Beach Diet Cookbook	*Dr Arthur Agatston*	£20
1-4050-3286-3	Stay Fertile Longer	*Mary Kittel*	£12.99
1-4050-3340-1	When Your Body Gets the Blues	*Marie-Annette Brown and Jo Robinson*	£10.99
1-4050-7330-1	The Women's Health Bible	*The Editors of* Prevention	£14.99

All Pan Macmillan titles can be ordered from our website, *www.panmacmillan.com,* or from your local bookshop and are also available by post from:

Bookpost, PO Box 29, Douglas, Isle of Man IM99 1BQ
Tel: 01624 677237; fax: 01624 670923; e-mail: *bookshop@enterprise.net*; or visit:
www.bookpost.co.uk. Credit cards accepted. Free postage and packing in the United Kingdom

Prices shown above were correct at time of going to press.

Pan Macmillan reserve the right to show new retail prices on covers which may differ from those previously advertised in the text or elsewhere.

For information about buying *Rodale* titles in **Australia,** contact Pan Macmillan Australia. Tel: 1300 135 113; fax: 1300 135 103; e-mail: *customer.service@macmillan.com.au*; or visit: *www.panmacmillan.com.au*

For information about buying *Rodale* titles in **New Zealand,** contact Macmillan Publishers New Zealand Limited. Tel: (09) 414 0356; fax: (09) 414 0352;
e-mail: *lyn@macmillan.co.nz*; or visit: *www.macmillan.co.nz*

For information about buying *Rodale* titles in **South Africa,** contact Pan Macmillan South Africa. Tel: (011) 325 5220; fax: (011) 325 5225; e-mail: *roshni@panmacmillan.co.za*

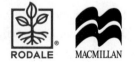

RODALE MACMILLAN